ASPIA's

Handbook

for

Partner Support

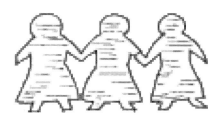

A collection of ASPIA's best information

for the support of partners

of adults with Asperger's Syndrome

Written / Compiled by Carol Grigg

Co-Founder and Co-Ordinator of ASPIA

(Asperger Syndrome Partner Information Australia Inc)

Copyright

ASPIA's Handbook for Partner Support
A Collection of ASPIA's best information for the support of
Partners of adults with Asperger's Syndrome

Paperback, First Edition 2nd Revision

ASPIA's Handbook for Partner Support is also available as an eBook from the following link:
http://www.lulu.com/content/e-book/aspias-handbook-for-partner-support/12936851

http://www.lulu.com

About this Book

Asperger Syndrome Partner Information Australia Incorporated (ASPIA Inc) is a Sydney-based support group for partners of adults with Asperger's Syndrome.

This book, which we have called ASPIA's Handbook for Partner Support, is a collection of ASPIA's best information gathered since our founding activities in the year 2000 right through to the present.

Feedback has confirmed over and over again that information is vital to understanding, and understanding is the key element making a difference in countless relationships and homes all around the world.

Through ASPIA, many partners have finally found the explanations they needed to make sense of their relationship bewilderment and take a more realistic and constructive approach towards the future.

By sharing the material in this book we are hoping that many more partners from around the world can benefit from the shared understanding and ideas of hundreds of partners who've attended our meetings and the wonderful education and support that ASPIA has received from several passionate psychologists in Sydney, as well as the ever faithful Tony Attwood from Brisbane.

Carol Grigg, April 2012

ASPIA's Handbook for Partner Support

TABLE OF CONTENTS

Section 5 Words fail us – Advocacy and Representation 93

Section 1 The Journey Begins

ASPIA: A Place for Validation, Information, Inspiration

ASPIA INC

A place for . . .

. . . Validation

        . . . Information

                . . . Inspiration

Mutual acknowledgement and understanding of the Asperger marriage experience for partners of adults with (or suspected of having) Asperger's Syndrome.

ASPIA's Commitment

"Most partners contacting ASPIA for support are deeply motivated to save the relationship that they have spent so long investing in and being part of, therefore ASPIA's commitment remains to continue to provide validation, information and support for as long into the future as is possible".

Carol Grigg, March 2012.

Why write this book?

The idea for providing a handbook for partner support grew out of our own ongoing search for realistic and reliable information that we could pass on to partners through our support group meetings and also our website. After conducting monthly support group meetings in Sydney, Australia since 2003, and establishing the website www.aspia.org.au in 2005, feedback has confirmed over and over again that information is vital to understanding, and understanding is the key element making a difference in countless relationships and homes all around the world.

This book, which we have called ASPIA's Handbook for Partner Support, is a collection of ASPIA's best information gathered since our founding activities in the year 2000 right through to the present.

Partners who attend our monthly meetings are nourished by the sharing of combined experiences and wisdom that have been gathered from the contributions of hundreds of partners who've attended over the years, and also the solid and consistent education provided by our favourite psychologists who are acknowledged on the following pages.

ASPIA's library contains many great books too that have fed us with the insights and perspectives of wise authors who've walked our journey, both in Australia and overseas.

Our Handbook for Partner Support also includes some additional information written and used in ASPIA meetings that may be useful as a model for those who'd like to establish a partner support group or conduct support work with partners. Having been operating consistently now since June 2003, we have had time to track the group experience and also the experiences of many partners attending our group, helping us know what works in the group and what doesn't. As a result ASPIA continues to conduct stable and successful monthly meetings and to make a difference in the lives of those individuals who we are blessed to be able to support.

For me, I feel deeply privileged to have been present when partner support was just in its early days internationally, and then during every moment of our own group's story since its earliest beginnings in Sydney. My passion for partner support has been inspiring my pen now for many years as I seek to describe and interpret this hidden world that partners share, and it is my desire that by compiling my own writings and ASPIA's best information into a handbook more partners around the world can benefit from a realistic, comprehensive and compassionate guide for their journey.

Permission is given for the information in this handbook to be reproduced for the purpose of partner support, provided each article, item or list is reproduced in full with clear acknowledgement of ASPIA and/or Carol Grigg as the source or author, and inclusion of ASPIA's website address www.aspia.org.au .

Our best wishes to every partner, professional or group leader who reads and uses this guide to inform, validate and inspire their own experience and help others on the journey along the way.

Carol Grigg, Co-Founder & Co-Ordinator, ASPIA INC, Asperger Syndrome Partner Information Australia Incorporated.

Acknowledgements

Since our beginnings ASPIA has been privileged to receive regular education and support from a number of very qualified and experienced professionals who are passionately devoted to understanding Asperger's Syndrome and supporting people affected by it including partners, children and family members.

The strength, stability and effectiveness of ASPIA's support work has been greatly influenced and undergirded by these psychologists, who we would like to acknowledge and thank here:

Lydia Fegan (Sydney, now retired)

Tony Attwood (Brisbane)

Jeroen Decates (Sydney)

Eleanor Gittins (Sydney)

Julie Peterson (Sydney)

A number of information sheets or lists provided in this handbook contain direct comments and suggestions provided by these psychologists during workshops, meetings or discussion groups, and have been repeated with their knowledge and permission, for which we thank them on behalf of partners all around the world.

A great deal of other information in this book also represents the depth of understanding and growth that has taken place in the hearts and minds of partners as a direct result of ASPIA's support, also resulting from the education provided by these wise and insightful psychologists and a number of other supportive professionals and authors along the way.

Contact details for these and other recommended professionals or organisations are on ASPIA's website, as well as a list of books & recommended authors.

About the Author

Emerging from 20 years of marriage to a husband with Asperger's Syndrome, and parenting five children within that environment, Carol has gone on to co-found and co-ordinate ASPIA, a support group and website for partners of adults with Asperger's Syndrome based in Sydney.

The passion that drives her is based on the desperate isolation and lack of support that eventually contributed to her own family's collapse, and the awareness that this is still happening to families today.

It is Carol's firm belief that many of these families can survive and even thrive if the Asperger characteristics are recognized in an individual or family when they present for professional help and if appropriate information and supports can be provided in a timely and sensitive manner.

Introduction to Partner Support

As fast as children are being diagnosed with Asperger's Syndrome, so are many adults being identified with characteristics of the same, often following the diagnosis of a child in the family. Sometimes there may not appear to be any family link, although it is commonly noted that the characteristics of Asperger's Syndrome do seem to run in families.

It is typically accepted that the diagnosis of an Autism Spectrum Disorder in a child is a crisis for any family. For the child, as one considers the difficulties they will face socially, in their educational pathway and their relationships into the future. For the family, as its role must change to take on greater support and intervention responsibilities than previously expected, and often they do this without adequate information, resources or professional, family or community support. Emotional and physical energy is challenged to the extreme as adjustments are made to family roles and daily life as well as hopes and expectations for the future.

It follows then that the identification or diagnosis of Asperger traits in an adult will also be experienced as a crisis within an affected family. For the adult, the crisis can be the stigma of being "different" that a diagnosis brings, and then the fear of discrimination and rejection that may follow, particularly while they grapple to understand just what the diagnosis means. For many the diagnosis does eventually, and even sometimes instantly bring relief as they finally understand the reasons why they have felt "different" for much of their lives. The diagnosis can release them to finally understand, accept and embrace themselves for who they are and recognize that the special abilities and gifts they possess are also as a result of having Asperger's Syndrome. For many, these gifts may have brought them success in their academic or vocational world, or provided a refuge in which to soothe away the stresses of life's relentless expectations. For others however, the struggle has been consistently difficult, and the diagnosis may not be met with the same optimism or relief, although it is encouraging to note that appropriate supports and interventions can make an enormous difference. Often self-acceptance leads to social acceptance as an adult with Asperger's Syndrome learns to be realistic about their difficulties.

The crisis that partners or family members will face involves the acceptance that the puzzling need for additional support and adaptation around the family member with Asperger's Syndrome will continue. Partners and family members have typically been aware for a very long time that there is something different about the adult with Asperger's Syndrome, and that there are a significant number of situations within the family context being affected adversely by some unexplained factor which has never been identified, managed well or resolved. It is discouraging to accept that diagnosis will not necessarily enable these difficult situations to be overcome, but encouraging to know however that better management may be possible in time, as a thorough knowledge is gained by each family member, including the adult with Asperger's Syndrome. It will however be necessary for the relationships and family situation to continue to be adapted to accommodate the differences that Asperger's Syndrome introduces.

For some partners and family members, accepting that ongoing support and adaptation will continue as a necessary part of family life into the future is all but too much. Sadly, the lack of knowledge and support has taken too great a toll on the human frame and heart for too long, and there is no energy, courage or resolve left to recover and re-build on the new foundation of awareness and knowledge.

The existence and ongoing success of ASPIA and other support groups and forums bears testimony to the continuing need for information and support for partners and family members in these challenging family situations. Typically it appears to be the non-Asperger partners or family members who embrace the need to pursue knowledge and professional support in order to give the relationship or family situation the best chance at surviving and even thriving. Sadly, often as a result of deficits in self-awareness and insight, and sometimes because of a desire to "save face" the typical response of the partner or family member with Asperger's Syndrome is to avoid or deny that there is any problem or to refuse to co-operate wholeheartedly with professional guidance. This leaves the burden of the relationship responsibility wholly on the non-Asperger partner or family members which is unworkable in any fulfilling way.

Long term support group experience does indicate however that in situations where the partner with Asperger's Syndrome is willing to accept the presence of traits, learn as much as they can about managing the traits in the context of relationships and family life and co-operate with attempts to improve the relationship difficulties, the non-Asperger partner or family member is encouraged and relieved and will meet the efforts with renewed energy and commitment.

Most partners contacting ASPIA for support are deeply motivated to save the relationship that they have spent so long investing in and being part of, therefore ASPIA's commitment remains to continue to provide validation, information and support for as long into the future as is possible.

Hearing and acknowledging people's stories and personal truth provides all-important validation. Without validation no partner can find a place to begin the journey of healing and recovery. Without identification with others in similar situations, no partner can recover a sense of self and worth. Without information and education no partner can come to a place of understanding the differences of Asperger's Syndrome and the ways it has affected the relationship. Without support no partner can sustain the courage and energy required to continue the journey. Without inspiration no partner can hold on to hope that better days may lie ahead.

For so long we've walked alone without understanding why. Now we know, and we pray for the strength and courage we need to continue the journey towards the hope that we've never wanted to relinquish.

Carol Grigg, 26 March 2012

Disclaimer

ASPIA is a support group and information source for those who are involved in or interested in marriage and long-term relationships with adults with Asperger's Syndrome (or suspected of having Asperger's Syndrome).

At no time has ASPIA claimed, nor does ASPIA claim, to be providing professional advice to its members and enquirers.

Whilst all care is taken to share information from reliable sources, ASPIA does not take responsibility for the way this information is implemented in personal situations.

At all times ASPIA encourages partners and other affected individuals to seek professional advice relevant to their individual situation from a qualified practitioner such as a psychologist, psychiatrist or counsellor. Dated: 29 July 2005

Section 2 The Legacy of Ignorance

Those Years without Light

"Asperger Syndrome will affect some of the fundamental ingredients required for relationships either to form or to be maintained. Sometimes relationships may struggle on for years in the belief that it will get better with time. Yet, in an intimate relationship, for example, neither of the couple is aware of what is causing the problems and persistent misunderstandings. This can wear down the mental and physical health of both and affect their self-esteem."

This comment has been quoted from Maxine Aston's "Asperger Couple Workbook".

Validation is Essential

Whilst some of the information in this section may now be "dated", covering the early days of Asperger awareness and a decade-long era of incomplete understanding, there has still been an important story emerging that needs to be told, and needs to be remembered for the validating benefit it can provide for those who lived for many decades of their lives without the knowledge they needed on a daily basis to cope and respond appropriately to partners and family members who subsequently have been identified as having the characteristics of Asperger's Syndrome.

"In a just and humane society, there needs to be space for everyone's story to be told." (Quote from Seasons for Growth learning materials, see www.goodgrief.org.au)

ASPIA would like to acknowledge here that every individual with Asperger's Syndrome also needs to benefit from an opportunity to tell their story, and to have their personal experiences of confusion and difficulty acknowledged. It is wonderful that many organisations now exist that can provide this validation, as well as the ongoing support they deserve.

ASPIA was established to provide an opportunity for partners of adults with Asperger's Syndrome to receive the much-needed validation they also deserve. ASPIA quickly recognized though that whilst validation is extremely important it is not enough on its own, and needs to be coupled with solid and reliable information, education and professional support. For almost a decade now ASPIA has sought to provide opportunities for validation, education and professional referral for partners who seek our help.

The beginning of every partner's journey of discovery must be met with validation of their story, their truth. This is the only pathway out of the confusion. As the story is told, it is met with affirmation and explanation. This is where understanding begins. Understanding brings the possibility of healing, forgiveness and hope.

It is essential that the story of partner experience is told in these pages, and it is ASPIA's absolute belief that the validation these pages bring will define a starting point for the journey forward.

"There is no greater agony than bearing an untold story inside you." (Maya Angelou, also from Seasons for Growth learning materials)

Carol Grigg, March 2012

Poem: My Asperger Marriage

From the beginning an awareness that something is wrong

A relationship that's fundamentally flawed and limited

Intimacy eludes every effort

Subconscious grief

Cold reality slowly settles in my heart

A loneliness that shouldn't be

A relationship that consumes every facit of my being

Yet abandons my basic human need to belong

Controlled, yet abandoned

Dominated, yet neglected

Needed, yet no-one

Promised, yet nothing

Diagnosis acknowledges what I already know

It is everything I thought, yet more

Blackness engulfs my soul like a shadow with form

Crushing out every whisper of hope

Or anticipation of something better

At first a relief

A book of answers for decades of questions

Reassurance of my own sound state of mind

Acknowledgement of all the hard work and pain

Just keeping it all on track

No healing, no solution, no remedy

A new way to live

A new way to love

New rules for ordinary things

Strategies for daily functioning

Mechanical methods

Altered responses

For better or for worse, in sickness and in health

All of these, all at once

A different state of being

A different definition of marriage

Bound, but alone

Alongside, but solitary

The sense of loss is engulfing

Loss of hope

Loss of dreams

Grief for what will never be

No union of two free minds and souls

Bound in love, care & respect

It's not like that and never will be

One free mind

One with sharp corners

One soul that lives & breathes with love and spontaneity

One that calculates & orders, hides, fears and rages

No effort on my part can change his state of mind

My love doesn't warm him

My care doesn't reach him

My personality doesn't win him

My feelings and opinions don't sway him

A different life

Carol, 14 December 2002

Poem: The Hidden Face

Asperger's Syndrome
What does this mean?
So few have heard
Fewer understand
How can I define it?
What is it like?
Once words are applied
Meaning seems so lost

Behaviours kept secret
For the world that he shares
With wife and child only?
How can this be?
Real, yet intangible
Unseen by others
How we seem like liars
Bitter, neurotic

Uncertain, incredible
Blamed, demoralised
Yet I am the backbone
Why would anyone believe me?
I look for your assent
You must tell me it is true
But you can't see it happening
To you it is not real

He seems so clear,
So certain, so adamant
No need for compromise
His way is best
His opinions correct
They have to be

Or why would he possess them?
Somehow I believe him

But I know …
Something's not right
How can I be sure?
How can I find help?
When those who do listen
Only pity and placate
Look after yourself
All men are like that

Intellectual, gifted,
So verbal and self-assured
A guide, we thought
For a life of purpose and drive
Clear cut values
Strong morals too
Admirable principles
Interesting views
Activities and interests
Show competence and skill
Loyal, faithful
Committed to a cause

Yet it seems like a façade
So perfectly worn
For when we go home
He's nowhere to be seen

Just somebody there
Who looks quite the same
But sounding so different
He looks at me strange
Misunderstanding, getting angry

Taking tangents when we talk
Where did it start?
Will it ever be resolved?

Where is the truth?
His logic is not mine
My words carefully chosen
Don't mean what they do
He resists my requests
He questions my needs
He loses touch
A disconnected world

Things seemingly trivial
Matter so much to him
His children are afraid
Not sure what he'll do
Yet he misses the point
That we need him so much
We need him to love us
To be gentle but strong

To care and show empathy
Mutual understanding, support
But it all goes wrong
We do what we can
But to him it means something else
His competence under fire
Every comment I make
Is a personal attack

Some friends find him brash
Intrusive, tactless, cold
I try to explain
Smooth it over

Mend the rift

I feel ashamed

Though his rudeness disconcerts

Belief in my tale still isn't won

His words cut like glass

Shattering in my wounds

My motives misunderstood

My love misconstrued

My spirit is broken

My strength nearly gone

Like a strangler fig vine

Asperger's Syndrome consumes my being

Till I wither . . .

Carol

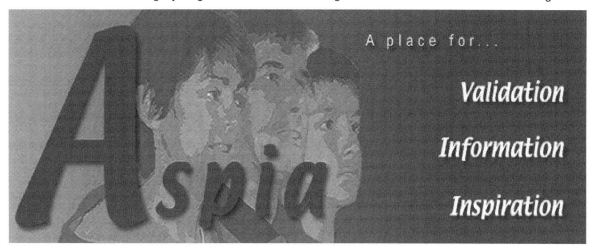

ASPIA Marriage Brochure

Asperger's Syndrome in Marriage (Aspia's Marriage Brochure © ASPIA 2006)

Over the last decade many people would be aware that there has been an upsurge of awareness and diagnosis of Autism and Asperger's Syndrome. Most of the cases being identified are children. Their behaviours are often exposed and uninhibited, allowing for ready identification and appropriate intervention and assistance to take place. Improved behaviour& communication patterns in turn enable more successful adjustment into adulthood.

What many people will not be aware of is that there is a second wave of identification taking place within the adult population. For adults with Asperger's Syndrome, their behaviours since childhood have gone "underground" and layers of coping strategies and defence mechanisms greet the social world. These behaviours often give the impression of someone quite "together" - perhaps a little eccentric or odd -but passable because of their high intelligence, impressive knowledge, high integrity and particular flair or gift in an area or career, such as engineering, telecommunications, computers, art, religion, politics, etc.

Many adults with Asperger's Syndrome do marry and have children. Marriage often follows a period of "ideal" courtship. However the experience of the partners and children are quite different to what most partners would experience and expect. Partners of an adult with Asperger's Syndrome often have awareness early in the marriage that something is not right but they can't work out what. They often speak of being aware that something, like a piece of a puzzle, is missing.

Partners with Asperger's Syndrome (AS)

The partner with Asperger's Syndrome can manifest a wide range of varying behaviours with varying intensities. However feedback from their partners in marriage suggests there are many common threads in their experience of marriage.

Below is a list of some common characteristics of the marriage experience and of the partner with Asperger's Syndrome, as described by members of the ASPIA Partner Support Group:

- An essential need to have things done in a prescribed manner or order.
- A tendency to correct and instruct those around them.

- Seeming to be experiencing "normal" situations differently, noticing different things and having to deal with different priorities which often prevent co-operation and teamwork, leading to frequent conflict. As a result the relationship and communication deteriorate quickly. Efforts to reason and resolve situations often result in partners feeling that they have been dug in deeper. They often feel that their efforts have been fruitless and even worse, have increased the level of complication.
- Verbal combat around "technicalities" or "order" of a situation rather than the "spirit" or "essence".
- Apparent evidence that the partner with Asperger's Syndrome is not "reading" situations or people intuitively and is consequently behaving insensitively or inappropriately for the circumstances.
- The partner with Asperger's Syndrome may appear to have an air of superiority or even arrogance and an apparent lack of respect for the knowledge, credibility, expertise or authority of others. They may have high intelligence or gifted abilities in some areas but seem to lack basic "common sense" or "know-how" in other more commonplace situations.
- The partner with Asperger's Syndrome may not recognise the effort their partner is constantly contributing to the relationship to try to sustain it. They may be extremely sensitive and easily upset, and may take issue or be offended over small matters which in turn can seem to jeopardize the stability or quality of the whole relationship.
- Interests and hobbies of some partners with AS tend to take on an obsessive characteristic at the expense of all other needs, duties and relationships around them.
- There is frequently a tendency to hostility, defensiveness and retaliation if the partner with Asperger's Syndrome is challenged or thwarted.
- The partner with AS can behave intrusively.
- They may be very controlling.
- The partner with AS may take roles seriously, to the letter of the law, especially as "Head of the Home" in a family with religious beliefs or tendency to traditional roles.
- Their courtship style is almost "too good to be true".
- After marriage the partner with AS often seems to lose motivation to keep working on the quality of the relationship as though the wedding day has "completed" their pursuit, allowing them to pursue other interests.
- The spouses of partners with AS claim that their spouses often do not appear to read the needs or notice the emotions of other family members, and they don't enquire or reach out to them. However, when they do notice a need or "we tell them about our needs, they don't seem to know instinctively what to do to make us feel better, and they will often do nothing and remain disconnected".
- The partner with AS may have great difficulty co-operating with others or working as part of a team or unit. They may seem focused only on what's going on for them, and unaware of what's going on for those around them.
- They often seem to over-react to efforts to talk over matters with them and may perceive such efforts as a personal attack.
- They often have difficulty coping or adapting around the daily "happenings" within a family situation.
- They may insist on predictability in others and in household activities, but seem to "live on a whim" themselves, leaving the family feeling uncertain all the time.
- The partner with AS may "shut-down" if they don't know what to say or how to behave. They may disengage with partner or family indefinitely.

- They may also "melt-down" or have episodes of rage and aggression when they don't know how to deal with circumstances, or they don't want to discuss, negotiate, compromise or resolve situations.
- They may hold to a single method or opinion in many areas of daily life.
- Social isolation may result for the family if the partner with AS is consistently avoiding social situations. On the other hand, some partners with AS can seem like the "life of the party" and keep everyone entertained or "engaged" (willingly or unwillingly) by sharing a great deal of expert knowledge on favourite topics of interest.
- The partners of people with AS will often feel as though they should and need to "repair" social faux pars, etc created by Asperger partner.
- Some partners with AS may be very controlling and unjust with the use of family finances, or on the other hand, avoid any financial responsibility within the household completely. They can quickly run the family into financial crisis by spending excessively on special interests, collections or hobbies.

Parenting

- If a parent with Asperger's Syndrome chooses to take an interest in their child they can be very attentive and go to great lengths to assist them in practical ways.
- On the other hand, they may have trouble reading their child's needs or emotional state and may either respond inappropriately or not at all, leading to the possibility of neglect or mishandling.
- They may not always be aware of or anticipate situations of danger or neglect when caring for a child.

The Experience of the Non-Asperger Partner

Partners living in a marriage or long-term relationship with an adult with Asperger's Syndrome report feeling a deep impact on their lives in the following ways:

- Confusion
- Frustration
- Powerlessness
- Isolation
- Being disbelieved by others, including professionals
- Burn-out
- Sense of being a mediator and interpreter at home and outside the home
- Loss of sense of self
- Changes in personality in order to cope with AS partner's behaviour
- Increase in feelings of anger
- Feeling like partner won't cope without them (if we separate)
- Trapped
- Shouldering responsibility for most household matters and well-being
- Neglected emotionally
- Constantly criticized and blamed unreasonably
- Alone
- Like a single parent
- Often feel in damage control or crisis management.
- Hyper vigilance to prevent chaos and relationship breakdowns
- Verbally, psychologically and sometimes physically abused
- Efforts to build and sustain relationship constantly sabotaged by pedantic requirements of AS person.

- Depression
- Hopefulness dashed
- Sense of sadness at unrealised potential in themselves, AS partner and other family members
- Unsupported
- Often betrayed by lack of loyalty and kindness from AS partner

The Benefits of Attending a Support Group

- Being with others who "know"
- Validation of our experiences
- No need to explain, prove or justify ourselves or our experiences
- Reassurance of our own worth and sanity
- No longer alone
- Opportunity to gain more understanding of Asperger's Syndrome.
- Regular opportunities to hear professionals speak.
- Information and feedback about other helpful services and professionals.
- Learn strategies to help us cope and manage better.
- Help us heal.
- Special Events give us opportunity to promote awareness of, and learn more about Asperger's Syndrome.

ASPIA stands for Asperger Syndrome Partner Information Australia. ASPIA is a support group and information source for partners of adults with Asperger's Syndrome. We commenced meetings in June 2003 (under our former name "GRASP").

The information we provide is not only helpful for partners, but also for anyone interested in understanding Asperger's Syndrome in adults and relationships in general.

Our Partner Support Meetings are held from 2pm – 5pm on the first Saturday of every month (except January) at The College of Nursing, 14 Railway Parade, Burwood, NSW. ASPIA contact details and enquiries: PO Box 57 Macarthur Square LPO, MACARTHUR NSW 2560. Ph: 0432 507 828 www.aspia.org.au

Asperger's Syndrome in Marriage, Helpful Explanations and Information for the non-Asperger Partner (original Spouse Workshop notes from 2001)

Helpful Explanations and Information for the Non-Asperger Partner

The following notes comprise official notes by Psychologist Tony Attwood and personal notes of the writer taken down during "Workshop for the Partner of a Person with Asperger's Syndrome" held in Brisbane, Queensland (Australia) on Saturday 25 August, 2001.

The notes have been re-arranged & grouped by topic to assist with ease of reading and reference.

Males outnumber females with Asperger's Syndrome, therefore "he" or "him" is used throughout this document.

WHY I WOULD HAVE BEEN ATTRACTED TO MY ASPERGER PARTNER

- Admiration for his intellect & abilities
- Compassion for his limited social skills
- Belief that his character was due to his childhood circumstances & that he will change in new relationship.
- Shared interests
- The degree of his adulation for me
- His fidelity or uprightness in relationships
- Pillar of community or similar
- Creative in their work with good career prospects
- Similar characteristics to my father in some ways

WHY HE WOULD HAVE CHOSEN ME

- He would instinctively have chosen someone with a similar profile of abilities as himself or a carer type with opposite characteristics
- Need for a replacement mother
- Will more often seek out a maternal type
- Dominant/submissive relationship will be essential
- Partner is usually maternal and loyal

GOOD QUALITIES OF AN ASPIE

- Ability in their career or special interest area
- Attention to detail
- Will speak their mind & are determined to speak the truth
- Their agenda will be obvious
- Advanced vocabulary & knowledge
- Unique perspective in problem solving (lateral thinking)
- Exceptional memory for detail
- Sense of social justice
- Practical in issues of mortality & grief

NEGATIVE SIDE OF GOOD QUALITIES WHEN APPLICABLE TO A RELATIONSHIP

- Special interest area may be an obsession & take over
- Pedantic in attention to detail & justice
- When speaking their mind will be tactless
- Determination to speak the truth will be more important than people's feelings
- Can't mask or hide their agenda
- Advanced vocabulary & knowledge may only apply to specific, favourite areas of interest & they will tend to dominate social & relational settings with these topics
- Problem solving techniques can be a real asset in practical areas but not when applied to emotions & relationships as the tendency is to reduce these to practical strategies
- Memory for detail can be useful
- Sense of justice can be tedious because of the need to reduce relationship to rules & equality
- Practicality in issues of mortality & grief can mean they have very short-lived emotion or none at all.

FURTHER NEGATIVES IN RELATIONSHIPS

- Two-way misinterpretation of signals between themselves & others
- Offensive to others by their blunt honesty
- Communication is just an exchange of information not a conversation
- They can pretend to be normal
- They prefer isolation
- Black & white in friendships
- May view "touch" as suggestive of sex
- May disclose personal matters inappropriately
- Difficulty relating on an emotional level
- Patterns in relationships may follow exact situations from books
- Understands objects more than people
- Will be unconventional because of different priorities & personal rules
- Need to have their own way
- May act like a teenager
- Has his own agenda
- May display arrogance & denial
- May have low self-esteem & depression
- Will be impulsive & reactive; he may know what to do but doesn't put it into practise because he doesn't think first
- They benefit from the flexibility & compassion of others
- Rigid in thinking – own ways of problem solving
- Unable to recognise when they're making a mistake & will think it's the thing or other people that are the problem.
- They create a structure around themselves in order to cope & can't change this.
- Denial of their difficulties
- Live in a world of action, not thought or emotion
- Don't see other people as being involved in the solution to their problems
- Will need to be reminded of the AS in order to keep his knowledge & awareness refreshed.
- Rarely apologise because they don't naturally admit wrong or recognise the need to feel better. May just be a "quick fix".

- Not self-reflective
- Differences in thinking seem like a severe cultural difference

EMOTION MANAGEMENT

- Mood swings (no brakes)
- Lacking an emotional toolbox – the ability to repair emotions
- Sudden intense rage (often over trivia)
- Emotion memory is short lived – he will tend to forget outbursts & want to move on while family/partner is still distressed
- May emotionally blackmail others

SPECIFIC DIFFICULTIES IN FAMILY LIVING

- Will have difficulty understanding natural childhood abilities & behaviour
- Rivalry with children
- Regimentation
- Problems with money management
- Special interest will take over
- They take on a "God" mode
- Paranoid
- Communication is an exchange of information, not a conversation
- High expectations of others
- Favouritism with children
- Needs it to be "my way"
- Critical of others
- Lack of affection & emotional support for children
- Intolerant of noise or mess but may be messy themselves
- Hoard items
- May have fundamental religious or political beliefs

DIFFICULTIES THE WIFE WILL FACE IN CONTEXT OF FAMILY LIVING

- Split loyalties between husband and children
- Acting as a diplomat
- In the firing line
- In reality is a solo parent
- In reality is mothering her husband
- Needs to be his executive secretary
- Aware of inequality in partnership
- Has to take care of social scripting – what to say, when & how to say it
- Has to repair & clean-up damaged relationships & social situations due to the havoc he leaves in his wake
- He will think he has said something when he has only thought it and be adamant he has said it
- He will think I should already know
- Dilemma of whether to go or stay
- Lives for "normal" children
- An AS child combined with AS father will reinforce each other against the wife/mother
- AS traits will be worse in times of change
- AS traits will worsen with more people around

- Life of uncertainty constantly wondering "Is it AS or is it normal?"
- Boys, either AS or NT, may model their father
- The problem components of family living are complex
- Husband always has his own agenda
- Wife's credibility will be irrelevant to AS husband
- He benefits from her flexibility & compassion which serves to reinforce his personal agenda
- He won't take wife seriously when she is "nice"
- She needs to be directive & blunt which goes against her nature
- Won't relate to emotive words, only logic
- Wife mothers him for the sake of the children & their relation ship with him
- Need to keep him aware of AS & its effect
- Even if divorced, wife would still have to arrange his visits with children
- Wife enables & facilitates his relationships, we bridge

MARRIAGE RELATIONSHIP & ROMANCE

- Special interest is his "mistress"
- In love with his special interest which brings him gratification on an intellectual level
- Communication is an exchange of information, not a conversation
- Wife is executive secretary
- Unequal relationship/partnership
- Wife takes care of social scripting & patching up havoc he leaves in his wake
- Two-way misinterpretation of signals
- "Touch" may be viewed by him as a signal for sex.
- Intimacy is limited in or absent of romance, seduction & foreplay
- Sex is an act, not an expression of love
- They may not even like being touched due to a tactile sensitivity
- Frequency & value of intimacy is limited & shallow
- Self-disclosure may be limited or non-existent on an emotional level
- Difficulty relating on an emotional level
- Behaviour may follow exact situations described in books
- Normal marriage counselling will be limited in effec-tiveness because they won't understand the importance of it or be able to put it into practise
- Not self-reflective
- He may indulge in multiple relationships & what's more, could expect his wife to be comfortable with this
- AS symptoms may strengthen in retirement or old age which leaves no escape for wife & no hope
- Wife has dilemma of whether to stay or leave but most of us stay because of our nature (maternal & loyal)
- Wife gives up own personality & sacrifices own life for him
- She lives for her children
- He will understand objects more than people
- AS traits worsen in times of change
- AS traits may worsen the larger the family
- AS partner will be the dominant partner because the NT partner will be more flexible
- NT partner will weigh up information in order to make a conventional decision whereas the AS partner will have different priorities & rules & they have to have their own way & this results in an "unconventional" decision.

- Life of constant uncertainty "Is it AS or is it normal?"
- Husband like a perpetual teenager
- Husband always has personal agenda
- Wife's credibility will be irrelevant to him
- He won't do things her way unless he wants to
- AS husband unable to fix emotions
- Won't respond when I ask in conventional "nice" ways
- Have to use logic rather than emotive words
- Wife is constantly blamed when things go wrong
- Has to cope with his denial of problem
- Wife mothers him
- Unable to ever leave emotionally, even if divorced
- Enabling & facilitating their relationships, even with us
- In divorce they would only recognise what can be quantified on paper in terms of property division, will not be able to recognise emotional value or input of parties involved
- Rarely apologise, only as a "quick fix"

SIGNIFICANT DISADVANTAGES FOR WIFE WHICH COMPOUND SITUATION

- AS husband doesn't recognise her credibility, it is irrelevant to him
- He is mostly in denial of problems
- Wife can't conceptualise to others what's going on
- Wife unable to convince others of the problem
- She is desperately in need of someone outside of family for back up, accountability for partner & to reinforce her credibility but almost impossible to obtain
- She gives up her own personality & life for him
- Unable to detach from him emotionally (maternal & loyal)

SPECIFIC NOTES ABOUT SPECIAL INTEREST

- May have great ability in area of special interest
- Special interest is their life, their achievement
- Understand objects more than people – often interest is technical, computers, model trains, science, knowledge of specific field, etc, etc.
- World consists of objects, knowledge & action (not thought or emotion)
- Can't separate the special interest from the AS
- Special interest gives them order, they define themselves by their objects around them
- Captured by the thrill of the chase, the planning and acquisition (this can apply to their acquisition of a wife too)
- Stopping them pursuing their special interest is like cutting off their arm
- Criticising his interest is like criticising him
- Pursuit of special interest becomes more compelling when stress levels rise
- May even break the law because special interest is so irresistible
- Operates according to his own agenda
- He is actually in love with his special interest & finds gratification from it on an intellectual level which may replace the need for physical gratification in relationship
- Special interest is their mistress
- Money management significant problem – excessiveness in special interest area but miserly in other areas

- Hoarding of items
- Fundamental religious or political beliefs may be involved

GENERAL SUGGESTIONS THAT MAY HELP

- Recognition of diagnosis – by partners & others
- Motivation of both partners to change & learn
- Support & contact with others in similar circumstances
- combined knowledge base & experience
- Support from other family members & own children
- Wife to have an independent social life
- Relationship counselling where Asperger Syndrome is understood by the counsellor
- Occasional escape for the wife
- A mutual understanding of the two different "cultures" and ways of thinking
- Emotion management strategies
- Guidance in social skills
- Open & effective communication
- External accountability (husband won't recognise wife's credibility)
- Division of household duties according to expertise
- Doing deals for reciprocal meeting of needs
- Wife needs to learn to be a bit "AS" back – blunt, straight, no negotiation, truthful, clear-cut, directive
- Wife needs to try & play the "AS" game
- Use logic, not emotive words
- Keep up with awareness & knowledge of AS by reading, etc

Compiled by Carol Grigg, ASPIA INC (Asperger Syndrome Partner Information Australia Inc)
www.aspia.org.au

Essay - Asperger's Syndrome in Adults and Families: The Tragedy of Late Diagnosis

Today we are living in a society where awareness and knowledge of Asperger's Syndrome is slowly but surely filtering through, and affected individuals and families are beginning to benefit from much more informed professional and community understanding and support. This is particularly so for those families who have a child with a diagnosis of Asperger's Syndrome.

Within the adult population however, society's lack of awareness of Asperger's Syndrome until the last 20 years has meant that many individuals, married couples and families have been experiencing significant impact in their lives from the characteristics of Asperger's Syndrome without having the opportunity of knowing what the underlying influence has been. Even today, very few professionals have enough knowledge and clinical experience of Asperger's Syndrome in adults to be able to recognize the subtle and often misleading indicators.

The characteristics and behaviours associated with Asperger's Syndrome in an adult can be difficult to recognize and often it is only the immediate family members who see and experience what others outside of the family don't see.

In an individual with Asperger's Syndrome, the Asperger characteristics will have been influencing their development from birth and will be entwined through the personality, temperament and every life experience.   In some individuals it may be more like a shadowing of characteristics rather than a diagnosable level, but still contributing enough to have an impact on the individual's primary relationships and social adaptability.

Just like any individual on this earth, individuals with Asperger's Syndrome will be psychologically affected by a whole range of childhood experiences which they may or may not have resolved over time. Due to differences in perception and difficulties with communication and social instinct, childhood experiences may have had a different impact on an individual with AS to that of a "typical" individual. Additional to this, their differences will have typically led to many confusing experiences of being misunderstood, rejected, bullied, punished, criticized, judged, disadvantaged, discriminated against and shamed, often quite unjustly.

Shamefully, society tends to be afraid or ashamed of, and therefore cruel, to those who are different, although I believe it is an important point to remember that society is made up of all types of people and not just those who are deemed to be "typical". People who are "different" themselves can often be guilty of rejecting or discriminating against those who they too perceive to be different. The acceptance of difference in self and others comes with knowledge, understanding, experience, love, self-awareness, humility and maturity.

When one considers the many challenges that people with Asperger's Syndrome must overcome every day just to meet societal demands, it is not hard to imagine and appreciate the level of courage and tenacity they must possess. Sometimes it is only within relationships, employment situations or times of crisis that the underlying difficulties surface, and affected individuals may not necessarily realize that they need help or know that they can approach a professional for help. Some have sought help, only to be misunderstood or misdiagnosed, and as a result of a very negative experience may never seek help again.

The awakening of awareness of Asperger's Syndrome within society has been leading to the discovery by many adults that someone they are in relationship with may be affected by Asperger's Syndrome. It may be their marital partner, one or both parents, adult child, sibling, close friend, colleague or other significant individual in their life. As will happen in any relationship where communication is hindered and difference is misunderstood, lack of awareness and understanding of Asperger's Syndrome will have led to a relationship being characterized by confusion, frustration, conflict, anxiety, grief, emotional distress and sometimes relationship breakdown. Considering that most of us are still seeking to resolve our negative childhood experiences and discover our own sense of self when we first marry, it is understandable that we will not be ready to manage the additional challenges that undiagnosed Asperger's Syndrome will contribute within a marital relationship.

If both individuals in a couple relationship are aware of Asperger's Syndrome, have a thorough understanding of how Asperger's Syndrome is affecting the individual and the relationship, are honest with each other, are mutually committed to finding solutions and have access to appropriate supports and professional help, there is no reason why a fulfilling partnership or relationship cannot be negotiated between an individual with Asperger's Syndrome and any other person.

Sadly, many individuals and couples have not had the benefit of information or support at crucial times of need in their life or relationship experience and are now struggling with the reality of personal or relationship breakdown.

Many adults affected by Asperger's Syndrome remain undiagnosed or in denial, and their partners are reaching out to find whatever information and support they can to help them understand, cope, recover their own sense of self, manage life better, influence improvement within the relationship and avoid divorce and legal conflict. Without the participation of the individual with Asperger's Syndrome in finding creative solutions for the relationship difficulties, the non-Asperger partner is left powerless to address key areas of conflict, or draw any emotional nourishment from within the relationship.

The establishment and rapid growth of partner support groups and online forums around the world is evidence of the grief, frustration and desperation that partners are experiencing as a result of the lack of timely information and support.

The growth of a massive online community of individuals with Asperger's Syndrome, who network through internet forums and blog sites, indicates that encouragingly there are many individuals with Asperger's Syndrome who have discovered the reason for their differences and difficulties and why they have struggled so much in certain areas throughout their lives. This discovery, with the internet as a medium, has enabled many of them to finally find the words to articulate their thoughts and experiences, to celebrate their gifts and abilities and to feel set free to find and fulfil their potential. Many have gone on to write books, establish organisations and websites, advocate, offer mentoring to help others with Asperger's Syndrome, or offer the world information on what Asperger's Syndrome is like from the inside. Their insight is invaluable to a world struggling to understand neurological difference and to discover effective approaches.

Many of these individuals then go on to explore the ways their Asperger characteristics may be impacting on the quality of their personal relationships with their partners, children, parents, other family members, colleagues and friends. Their honesty is to be commended and encouraged, and deeply welcomed by loved ones. Once an individual with Asperger's Syndrome can accept their differences and limitations and recognize their qualities and strengths, they are in a beautiful position to be able to work with the significant people in their lives to restore warmth, understanding and unity in whatever ways are possible.

Sadly, when individuals with Asperger's Syndrome remain in denial or refuse to honestly discover and accept their differences and difficulties, or take their own fair share of responsibility for relationship problems, then hope for renewed quality in their relationships will remain elusive and circumstances will continue to be bleak as misunderstandings and conflict continue unchecked.

When looking closely at the difficulties that occur in relationships affected by Asperger's Syndrome, one notes that a key characteristic that creates particular difficulty in relationship and family life is rigidity of thought and behaviour. This can often result in a tendency to make and enforce rules for ordinary, everyday things without an inbuilt flexibility or adaptability that provides for "on the spot" change/deviation or "spontaneous" alternatives that family life may demand or require. Instead, families report feeling rail-roaded, bullied or manipulated in some way into satisfying the Asperger individual's need for things to be done in a prescribed way. An individual with Asperger's Syndrome may use aggression to enforce their own method, or they may simply withdraw or refuse to "go along" with the family's preference. There are reasons for this that can be understood once one gains a thorough understanding of Asperger's Syndrome.

Families report feeling anxious about allowing household situations to develop that upset the person with Asperger's Syndrome and the experience of these families is that this can reduce family life to a system of systems, rules, roles, routines & formulas to ensure the predictability, order and "correctness" that the Asperger person seems to need in their life and environment to enable them to cope.

This need to impose order within family life does not necessarily carry through into the personal life of the individual with Asperger's Syndrome though, which creates further confusion for family members because of the perception of inconsistency or hypocrisy on the part of the person with Asperger's Syndrome. People with Asperger's Syndrome can in fact seem quite personally disorganised and may lack the "follow-through" necessary for attending to practical or financial responsibilities within the household. Once again there are reasons to explain this, once one understands AS.

Family members report that the Asperger individual comes across as seeming unusually self-focused and unable to acknowledge or demonstrate awareness of the individual thoughts, feelings, interests, preferences, abilities, stages and needs of other family members, which necessarily need to be incorporated into the daily functioning, flow and decisions of successful family life. As a result, family members can feel overshadowed, or not valued, included or appreciated for who they are. Some parents with Asperger's Syndrome have difficulty acknowledging achievements and ignoring failure, and may appear critical and hard to please. Sadly, some individuals with Asperger's Syndrome can tend to be quite aggressive, retaliatory or controlling in nature, and may regularly criticize, correct, put down or make condescending comments towards their partners or children, and sadly they may not display understanding or tolerance towards a child who may be different to other children in the family or who needs more attention or support. Out of frustration or intolerance, some parents may resort to physically abusive methods of discipline or restraint in order to maintain order and predictability or to bring certain behaviours or circumstances under control. Hopefully modern day attitudes and parenting approaches in the home will ensure that the present generation of children will not grow up with memories of this kind of treatment from any parent or caring figure. Many adults, Asperger or non-Asperger alike, carry deep and unresolved emotional pain from memories of this kind of treatment as a child from a trusted parental figure.

It helps for individuals with Asperger's Syndrome and family members to understand the role that anxiety may play in Asperger's Syndrome, and the way this can lead to certain behaviours and attitudes that would be defined as "controlling". It would seem to be common for people with Asperger's Syndrome to experience very high levels of anxiety, and to also develop significant defense mechanisms in order to help alleviate this anxiety, creating further complexity within a cocktail of difficulties.

It has been noted by families that an individual with Asperger's Syndrome within a family context can seem to come across as lacking insight into the impact that their attitudes, behaviours, words or withdrawal are having on family members and that they typically won't be open to feedback. Their tendency can be rather to blame the partner or child for causing the situation or being unjust in their claim or accusation. If there is an issue involving the handling of the children and the non-Asperger parent seeks to mediate, intervene or reason with the Asperger parent, the Asperger parent may withdraw or shutdown, or may react with aggression or accusation that the partner is attacking, criticizing or shaming them, or is against them.

As a result of these difficulties, the non-Asperger partner is left feeling confused and powerless, unable to effectively communicate or reason with the individual with AS, or bring about an improved perception of fairness for the children. A sense of fear, along with feelings of rejection and injustice begin to settle over family members.

It has been a common experience of partners and children that when they go outside of the home to seek help, their stories are frequently met with disbelief because, to the outside world, the characteristics of Asperger's Syndrome can remain so hidden, and the Asperger partner/parent may present as being competent, skilled and of upstanding character. In fact, the partner or child may be judged as being disturbed or holding unacceptable or malicious attitudes. Hence, the isolation is multiplied, which I understand also happens to those who report other forms of mistreatment taking place within a home or other situation. This leaves the non-Asperger parent in a situation where he/she cannot defend his/her children, secure help or find some form of accountability for the Asperger parent, or if it is a child seeking help, they are left vulnerable and isolated with no-one to advocate for them.

The matter of abuse is a very sensitive one, particularly in relation to Asperger's Syndrome. The majority of individuals with Asperger's Syndrome do not resort to deliberate acts of abuse or mistreatment against other individuals. The use of the word "abuse" in the context of this essay means "mistreatment" in some form, and not "mis-use". Families seeking information and support do report incidents of "abuse" within their homes, but in virtually every one of these incidents "abuse" would be defined as "mistreatment", not the"mis-use" of an individual or child for personal or sexual gratification. Family members do report feeling mistreated in verbal, emotional, mental, psychological and occasionally physical ways by the individual with Asperger's Syndrome. Whilst the "mistreatment" or "abuse" is not typically intentional or deliberate, the impact on family members is still emotionally damaging, the same as if it was intentional, and partners and children still find they need counselling to help resolve their feelings. In time, understanding of Asperger's Syndrome can help release blame and enable forgiveness and healing.

Sadly, all human beings are capable of abuse or mistreatment of others, particularly when we allow ourselves to express frustration in ways that harm or intimidate those around us. Asperger's Syndrome affects communication, and communication is the "tool" that every human being needs in order to be heard, understood, make our needs known, protect ourselves, navigate life successfully, nurture our relationships and resolve conflict. If the "tool" of communication is flawed or in disrepair, then individuals and their relationships can quickly fall into crisis.

An inability to effectively communicate creates enormous frustration, and most of us express frustration in ways that harm the very ones in our lives who rely on us for love and security.

Non-Asperger individuals are capable of expressing frustration in damaging ways and may at times emotionally escalate and react towards their Asperger partner in ways that are abusive. An individual with Asperger's Syndrome may have difficulty monitoring and managing their own internal emotions and frustrations, so may not have developed an adequate awareness of the impact their attitudes and behaviours are having on those around them. The possibility that their frustration could be expressed in ways that are harmful to others and therefore "abusive" is very real.

It is extremely important for families to realize that the "abuse" or "mistreatment" is typically inadvert and unintentional and can be understood by thoroughly understanding Asperger's Syndrome. A small minority of individuals with Asperger's Syndrome may learn to use certain "abusive" or aggressive behaviours deliberately to intimidate others or cause certain desired outcomes. Whilst Asperger's Syndrome can provide reasons for certain behaviours, it does not provide an excuse for mistreatment or abuse of any form, just the same as no individual on this earth can find justification for abuse or mistreatment of another human being.

The stories of many partners who've navigated a marital relationship and parenting with a partner with Asperger's Syndrome, sometimes for decades, indicate that lack of support and awareness of Asperger's Syndrome has led to them becoming frustrated, angry and bitter towards their partner with Asperger's Syndrome. They have not understood that it is a neurological difference that is influencing the communication difficulties and ability to resolve conflict. Instead, they have judged their partners as having poor character and having deliberately betrayed their trust, let them down, set them up to take advantage of them, blamed them for all the problems, controlled them or caused isolation purely for selfish reasons and hurt or neglected them emotionally. What the non-Asperger partner hasn't realized is that all along the partner with Asperger's Syndrome was struggling just to cope with life and the people around them, find the space they needed to restore calm to their inner being, avoid change or discomfort, create predictability and fill the roles that family or society has demanded of them.

It is fair to say however that every family affected by Asperger's Syndrome has had "normal" expectations of the Asperger parent because they have not been aware of or understood Asperger's Syndrome, and they have lived with deep confusion, frustration and emotional pain. What the family members experience can lead to long-term resentment towards the Asperger parent who is not understood, who is expected to be "normal", who is capable of creating a sense of fear and confusion within the family and who often seems unwilling to accept the opinions and feelings of family members. This can and often does lead to estrangement, and an adult child may make many attempts to reconcile with their Asperger parent over the passage of many years, even into old age, and yet fail to make progress or resolution with them, which is very sad.

It is vitally important to remember that Asperger's Syndrome is a neurological difference that changes the way people experience and relate to the world and other people. It is the realization of this truth that helps many family members to finally stop taking things personally and find emotional healing. Some people with Asperger's Syndrome can actually become very distressed in hind-sight when they realise that their partners, parents or children felt abused or mistreated by them. Sadly, in a small number of cases, the Asperger partner or parent appears not to care.

Family members who felt abused by an Asperger parent or family member and who can now view their past experiences through the "lens" of understanding of Asperger's Syndrome, can often find peace with their past and an ability to forgive, heal and move forward.

When partners finally come to understand the differences and difficulties that their Asperger partners have been challenged by, they are overwhelmed with grief, but also relief. They are relieved to realise that there has been a valid reason for all the confusion and conflict and that it wasn't them creating all the problems after all, even though their Asperger partners have often blamed them. They are relieved to learn that their AS partners are not of poor character, but that they have a neurological difference that affects communication, perception, social instincts and the ability to cope. The grief that overwhelms partners takes place as they re-live and re-evaluate every memory of relationship and family confusion and conflict and they realize that "if only" they had known sooner, they could have approached situations so differently and avoided so much harm and trauma to both partners and all family members.

For those families where the partner or parent with Asperger's Syndrome has accepted and embraced his or her own Asperger characteristics, who is being honest and is taking responsibility to manage any negative behaviours, then every member of that family can begin to embrace and celebrate their own individuality and work towards the realisation of their own potential.

As the awakening of awareness of Asperger's Syndrome within society continues, it is hoped that individuals with Asperger's Syndrome, their partners and their families can now finally be understood and offered the help and support they need in order to re-build their hopes, their relationships and the resilience and capacity they embarked on life with.

Partners and family members who are believed and supported can be the most supportive allies an Asperger adult can have. Understanding does make all the difference, and testimonials indicate that many partners and families are calmer, happier and managing much better as a result of receiving validation, information and support.

Written by Carol Grigg, September 2009, revised January 2012.

Carol Grigg is co-founder and co-ordinator of ASPIA INC, Asperger Syndrome Partner Information Australia Incorporated, which is based in Sydney, Australia. ASPIA has been conducting support group meetings since 2003 and established a website in 2005. It is estimated that several thousand partners or family members have approached ASPIA for information, support and referrals since 2003, and website statistics indicate that approximately 1400 people every week are reading information on ASPIA's website. Carol experienced 20 years of marriage, from 1983 to 2003, with a partner diagnosed with Asperger's Syndrome, and is the mother of five children. For more information about ASPIA or Asperger's Syndrome within marriage and families please visit ASPIA's website at www.aspia.org.au or email info@aspia.org.au .

Essay – When Divided Marriages became Divided Communities

I am writing this essay on behalf of many individuals world-wide who are members of groups for the support of partners of adults with Asperger's Syndrome.

Generally, and for the purpose of this essay, we shall call ourselves "Neurotypical" because we are deemed to be "neurologically typical" within society rather than "neurologically different" as are those who have Asperger's Syndrome, and as we believe our partners are, to a more or less degree.

I believe it is important to note here however that along the way on our own journeys of self-discovery some of us have uncovered the reality that we may also have some milder characteristics of Asperger's Syndrome. Generally, our partners appear to be demonstrating a much stronger degree of Asperger characteristics than we are, although they are typically very highly functioning adults in specific areas of life, particularly relating to academic and vocational achievements. Many of us have also given birth to children who are either Neurotypical, Asperger or Autistic or who display shadowing of Autism to a more or less degree. Asperger's Syndrome is indeed a family affair, and certainly a thing of degrees.

Due to the relatively recent discovery of Asperger's Syndrome (1990's), all of us, Asperger and Neurotypical, have been experiencing life and relationships without awareness and knowledge of Asperger's Syndrome. For some of us this has been long term – at least 10 years, many for 20 or 30 years, and some even more.

The message from the Asperger Community is that many of these marriages are successful and mutually satisfying. If we were able to learn from these couples, their experiences could form a vitally important resource for the rest of us who have experienced long-term confusing and complicated relationships where communication difficulties seem to be at the root of many of the complications.

Communication has many layers and components and is the essential tool required for forging and building relationships into understanding partnerships. Communication differences and difficulties have prevented many couples and families from being able to use the tool they needed to forge the mutually satisfying relationships they had envisaged.

Sadly, the lack of awareness of differing neurologies throughout our societies, for countless generations, means that all of us have contributed to a great deal of prejudice and abuse being perpetrated against those who are perceived as different or vulnerable. This lack of awareness combined with the selfish pride of the human heart has also prevented responsible efforts being made towards understanding those of different neurologies, and ensuring their inclusion, equality and empowerment within society. Of deep concern is that there is prejudice, hatred and inequality within our societies at all, and on personal reflection we know that all mankind is capable and guilty of these, regardless of our individual neurology.

The lack of awareness about differing neurologies, and in particular Asperger's Syndrome (being the focus of this essay) has sadly set up countless marital and family experiences of confusion, frustration and reaction down through many generations. With the discovery of Asperger's Syndrome and the hope this has brought, we are now all trying to find solid ground in the wake of what could be likened to a tsunami of misunderstanding created by generations of ignorance.

Without awareness of Asperger's Syndrome, or differing neurologies, no family member, Asperger or Neurotypical has known how to respond to the circumstances they find themselves in. Typically, none of us express our frustration in healthy ways and we've added abuse and shame to the confusion and frustration, thereby creating a sure formula for family destruction.

Our pride and the desperate determination to "save face" or "win" further builds up the wall between partners and family members, preventing us from backing down and loosening the tight grip we have on our own perspective. This is really fear. Fear of losing control. Fear of humiliation. Fear of being exploited. Fear of being blamed. Fear of financial disadvantage. Fear of being exposed. Fear of being alone. Fear of the unknown. And for many the fear is very real. Many partners, Asperger and even Neurotypical may exploit each other in relationships, may humiliate each other, may place blame on each other for the difficulties, may seek to financially control or gain financial advantage over the other, may hide from reality, avoid self-discovery, deny the ways they are damaging the relationship, refuse to accept accountability for their own actions, and sadly they may perpetrate abuse towards each other, verbally, psychologically and sometimes physically.

What has been happening in our marriages and family situations as described above, combined with the long-term confusion and sense of powerlessness, has fuelled deep anger, a sense of betrayal and increasing hostility. With the discovery of Asperger's Syndrome, there has been a flood of emotion and exuberance released and the anger and hostility we have been storing has unfortunately been carried forward and transferred into creating an arena of conflict and "them and us" mentality between the Neurotypical and Asperger Communities nationally and internationally, two previously undefined communities that have suddenly formed out of the destructive dust of our marriages. Awareness of Asperger's Syndrome has seemed to give form to what's been affecting our relationships. It is easy to then place all the blame on Asperger's Syndrome, when in reality Asperger's Syndrome describes the blockage or impedance in our ability to communicate. When communication is thwarted, couples are prevented from using the only tool they have available to them to develop mutual understanding and navigate life as a couple. No other issue in a relationship can be explored, unpacked, understood or resolved without effective communication.

Ideally, as is expressed in the words of a well-known leader within the Asperger Community, both communities now need to be "working to foster communication and understanding between equal partners with different methods of social communication".

It is our instinct that this is only possible once the differences between the two neurologies, ie Neurotypical and Asperger, are identified and understood. Then, equipped with this knowledge, the tool of communication is able to be formed and shaped in the way that will enable mutually meaningful communication to take place within each individual relationship. Then, and only then, can we begin to dismantle the walls built up between us, in our homes, in society and the communities that have emerged out of the world of cyber-forums.

What we have been witnessing is the formation of two separate seething communities creating stereotypes and generating hateful attitudes towards each other. We need to announce a "cease fire", put down our weapons and, without throwing out all the babies with the bathwater, use what we've learned to find ways to neutralise the hostility and defensiveness that exists within our personal relationships, and between our two communities.

Whilst the concept of "Cassandra" from earlier days has now become provocative, this concept has been useful to describe the voiceless and powerless existence of non-Asperger partners prior to the identification of Asperger's Syndrome in their situation.

Many have been seeking help and someone to hear them for years, sometimes decades, and have been disbelieved and left feeling demoralised, judged and shunned. This could also be true in the experience of someone with Asperger's Syndrome who's been aware of their difficulties and seeking help but has remained unheard, judged or misdiagnosed. Validation of one's experience is an extremely important first step essential to a successful journey forward. Once Cassandra's voice is heard however, and effective supports secured, she no longer needs to see herself as Cassandra. How thankful we are for the knowledge and support opportunities we now have, and the life-changing differences these are making for ourselves and our families.

Sadly, there is a legacy though, and for non-Asperger partners, this is what CADD (Cassandra Affective Deprivation Disorder) attempted to define. Partner support work has been largely pioneering work, uphill, difficult and very emotionally overwhelming. CADD was not meant to be used as a label for Neurotypical partners to remain stuck within, a fortress to remain safe behind or a weapon to be used to regain a sense of equality within the home, but as a starting place of validation for the journey of recovery, self-discovery and healing that becomes possible once the source of confusion and affront has been identified.

It is very likely that the partner with Asperger's Syndrome could also identify with similar steps and stages in their own journey. Discovery of their own Asperger characteristics must bring validation and relief, but the legacy of having lived without awareness of Asperger's Syndrome must leave a residue of depression and trauma that will require support and professional help for a successful journey forward.

Surely the legacy of depression and trauma that many of us carry with us, Neurotypical and Asperger both, has its origins in the lack of awareness of our differing neurologies, and the confusion and frustration we've experienced as a result of trying to conform to societal and marital "norms". Ah, the catastrophe this conformity has created. Thank God for the awareness we now have.

It is vitally important that Neurotypical partners and also people with Asperger's Syndrome derive their information and support from sources that are balanced and honest, where the equality, rights and value of every human being are upheld, where realities can be discussed with concern and compassion, and where no-one is verbally or emotionally bashed for their failings or their neurology. After a support encounter (groups, forums, etc), do we go back to our reality with a recovering sense of self, carrying some fresh ideas and hope, or do we go back to our reality feeling more angry and trapped? Good self-care will seek constructive support encounters.

Neurotypical partners do need help. We need help to understand our Asperger partners. We need help to know how to help re-build the communication bridge with our Asperger partners. We can't do it alone. Sadly, in the majority of Neurotypical/Asperger relationships our groups and forums represent, our Asperger partners are not participating, or only participating minimally. Unfortunately, this is what drives a lot of the negative sentiment that exists in the Neurotypical community.

A motto of a large international Asperger Support organisation is "Nothing about us, without us".

Our marriages are about both partners in a relationship, the partner with Asperger's Syndrome as well as the partner who does not have Asperger's Syndrome. The communities of Asperger and Neurotypical overlap by inter-marriage and pro-creation and we all need understanding and support in order to learn to communicate more effectively and prevent family breakdown wherever possible.

Both communities have a responsibility to the relationships their members have committed themselves to. We can make a difference, but only if the two communities, and both partners, find a way to work together.

We recognise that negative stereotyping has contributed to people with Asperger's Syndrome not wanting to identify as having AS, but with a positive campaign by the Autistic community aimed at de-mystifying AS, raising Autistic pride and providing relationship education for AS partners from an AS perspective, surely we can begin "working to foster communication and understanding between equal partners with different methods of social communication".

Carol Grigg, 2009 (revised 2012)

Essay – Injustice in the Family Court

A very sensitive and highly emotive issue in the Asperger Community has been the fear of unjust rulings within Family Court systems that could take place as a result of a parent bearing a diagnosis of Asperger's Syndrome, particularly as a result of the influence of certain claims being made by members of the non-Asperger community in relation to parenting by adults with Asperger's Syndrome.

It may be helpful to provide a little history or background to these matters involving the perception or fear of prejudice within the Family Court system that had been simmering within the Asperger community over a number of years to the point of eruption finally in 2009.

The original campaign began in the early 2000's and was driven by non-Asperger partners and parents concerned to contribute general awareness of Asperger's Syndrome to the legal system in an attempt to correct what was perceived to be a dangerous ignorance that could have led to dire consequences of disadvantage to any family member, either Typical or Asperger, adults or children, in families that find themselves the subject of a Family Court matter.

Several personal situations existed at that time where an Asperger partner/parent had a stronger verbal ability, more comprehensive knowledge of the law, greater eloquence, more financial resources, and more influence in the legal arena than their Neurotypical partners. This meant that whoever was able to prepare and present a more impressive "Case" won the Court hearing, regardless of that individual's history of actions, abilities or commitment within the family situation. Some individuals with Asperger's Syndrome at that time had been seemingly misrepresenting their performance, abilities and commitment within their marital and family situations. No avenue was made available through the Court in those cases for parental ability and commitment to be explored and assessed and for parents to be judged for their own actions. The Neurotypical partners/parents in these specific personal cases were somehow seen to have no credibility in comparison to the Asperger partner, and the concerns they raised were viewed as malicious or efforts at alienation rather than attempts to genuinely advocate for the best outcomes for their children, and indeed the whole family.

The original campaign for awareness was motivated by a desire to ensure that justice could take place for all, regardless of one's neurology, and not just those who could achieve an impressive representation in Court. A bias against any group of people based just upon their neurology was never the intention. The driving force was a need for awareness and education so that cases could be explored in fairness and truth and that justice could indeed be done, particularly for the innocent and powerless participants of any family situation – the children.

Unfortunately, the campaign to promote awareness of Asperger's Syndrome within the Court systems took on a fervour that led to a stereotyping of all people with Asperger's Syndrome as being abusive and unfit parents. This outcome was not the intention, only improved awareness and justice for all parties concerned was the desired outcome.

That any individual can receive a better outcome in Court based on their eloquence, financial capability or personal influence is a dark blot on any justice system anywhere. And that any individual can receive an unfavourable outcome based on their lack of eloquence, financial capability or personal influence is an even worse blot. It is likely that the Asperger community would have supported the original spirit of these endeavours.

It is to be hoped that now, in 2012, avenues have been found to promote awareness of Asperger's Syndrome within relationships and family situations in ways that encapsulate the needs and rights of all family members, whether Typical or Asperger, ensuring justice for all, especially the children.

Ideally, the best outcome is where responsibility is placed equally on both adult partners in a marital or family relationship to ensure, mutually, the well-being of the children they have conceived together and committed themselves to.

It is paramount that the Courts ensure that each case is thoroughly explored, without bias, to assess the capabilities and past performance of both parents, ensuring that the parent entrusted as primary carer of any child is the one that has demonstrated the most consistent and constructive family participation and not just the one that is best at preparing and representing a Case in a Court of Law.

I would suggest that the parent who has genuinely sought help, demonstrating transparency and a willingness to engage and co-operate with appropriate supports is most likely the parent who is most motivated and committed to ensuring the child's best interests as first priority.

Carol Grigg, 2009 (revised 2012)

Essay – Healing the Divide

Over the last ten years, growth of awareness of Asperger's Syndrome has led to the establishment and rapid growth of countless self-advocacy and support organisations for individuals with Asperger's Syndrome and their family members.

Individuals and families affected by Autism and Asperger's Syndrome need information and support, and derive great benefit from being able to identify with a community of people of shared experience.

These self-advocacy and support organisations provide opportunities for the voiceless to finally find a voice and a place to be heard.

Years and decades of hundreds of thousands of human experiences of confusion, bullying, abuse, victimisation, fear, anxiety, stress and grief tumble out of hearts, off the tongues and over the lips of those who claim to have Asperger's Syndrome, or to be a partner or family member of someone with Asperger's Syndrome. These experiences have been lived without awareness of Asperger's Syndrome, awareness that could have drastically altered the course of many lives for the better and prevented many devastating outcomes of personal and family breakdown.

Self-Advocacy and support organisations are vital for bringing information, understanding and supports into the lives of those who are struggling, and for building societal awareness and conscience in relation to attitudes and provision of appropriate services to individuals with Asperger's Syndrome and their families.

The collection of testimonials of partners and family members has led to the unhelpful creation of stereotypes that depict all individuals with Asperger's Syndrome as abusive, controlling, neglectful and emotionally harmful to those they are in relationship with. Family members speak of confusion, sadness, frustration, isolation, loss of hope, inability to cope, exhaustion, deep grief, family breakdown.

However, the testimonials of individuals with Asperger's Syndrome tell of relentless childhood abuse and bullying both at home and at school, disadvantage in employment, devastating misunderstandings and abuse within relationships and marriage, tremendous confusion and difficulty just facing social situations every day.

People from both groups tell of being disbelieved, brushed aside or unhelped by health care professionals, or of suffering years of incorrect diagnoses and treatments. Asperger's Syndrome can remain so hidden, and families and society remain so ignorant.

Advocates and leaders from both groups are emotionally weighed down by the testimonials that are shared with them, feeling a deep moral duty to speak up in defense of those they represent. Whilst testimonials may not count as official research or controlled studies, they are the voice of the people and cannot be ignored or denied.

But who will hear?

Without hearers, voices remain unheard.

Without understanding, difference continues to divide those who share homes and even beds.

Without advocacy, people with Asperger's Syndrome remain misunderstood, and without support, family members remain confused and isolated.

What is needed most and what can self-advocacy and support organisations ultimately hope to achieve, beyond hearing and supporting those they directly represent?

I would contend that our ultimate hope and goal should be to not just support the individuals we represent, but to play a part in influencing the development of mutual understanding and respect between the two groups, those who have Asperger's Syndrome and those who don't.

To make a positive difference in the homes and lives where difference has up until now created division, would have to be the ultimate hope that any advocate could hold.

Carol Grigg, July 2009, revised 2012

Essay – Are Asperger Marriages likely to be Abusive?

The issue of abuse in Asperger marriages and family situations has proven to be an extremely sensitive one, and it is fair to say that it is unfair to stereotype all people with the characteristics of Asperger's Syndrome as abusive, because they are not, although I do believe that certain aspects of Asperger's Syndrome do present a risk of inadvertent abuse within relationships unless these aspects are recognized and managed.

Defining Abuse

Before I write anything further I believe it is important to define what abuse is, particularly our meaning for the purpose of this article.

The main types of abuse in society are: physical, sexual, emotional, verbal, psychological, social, financial, mental and spiritual, as well as actions or omissions causing neglect or deprivation.

It is important to state that in this article I am not including sexual abuse in the meaning of the term "abuse". In the ten or eleven years that I have been listening to stories of families affected by Asperger's Syndrome, the reporting of sexual abuse appears to be virtually nil. This is not to say it doesn't happen, because the matter of sexual abuse is a particularly sensitive matter and not typically talked about lightly or with strangers, but I just don't have any grounds to suspect that this is common. It would seem possible however that a person with Asperger characteristics could on occasions behave inappropriately in a sexual way, but typically this is more likely to be inadvertent or unintentional.

It is fair to say that every person on this earth is guilty of some form of abuse towards others at some point in our lives, sometimes inadvertently, sometimes deliberately. None of us like to be accused of abuse however because of the shameful stigma associated with it.

On the other hand, most of us (non-Asperger and Asperger) have painful memories of having been abused at some stage in our lives, either in our developing years or within our relationships in adulthood, and by someone we trusted. The journey to find healing for ourselves and forgiveness for those who hurt us can be very painful and difficult, particularly when our abuser refuses to acknowledge the abuse or apologise for it.

There are many forms of abuse, but those of a sexual nature are particularly abhorrent leaving our hearts aching for those who have suffered abuse of this kind. The journey towards healing must be particularly painful and difficult for these ones. I re-iterate that in this article I am not referring to abuse of this nature, although I do not mean to deny that some readers may have experienced an awful violation such as this.

Abusive expressions or behaviours

Within the history of our partner support group, stories appear to indicate that individuals with Asperger's Syndrome do commonly express attitudes or behaviours that are experienced by their partners or family members as abusive in nature, whether inadvertent or deliberate. Typically these would be incidents of verbal, mental, emotional, psychological or social abuse, with some also experiencing some financial and/or spiritual abuse too. Most also report experiencing some form of neglect or deprivation by an adult partner, parent or family member with Asperger characteristics, though it is always important to stress that typically this will be inadvertent or unintentional.

It does make a huge difference for family members when they finally learn about Asperger's Syndrome and recognize the difficulties that people with Asperger's Syndrome have in social and relationship settings.

Abuse may be unintentional, but impact is the same as if intentional

Of course, we encourage understanding and accommodation as much as possible, but the fact remains that, even though any abusive attitudes and behaviours expressed by people with Asperger's Syndrome are typically unintentional, they are still experienced by the recipients as abusive in nature because of what those behaviours are typically thought to mean, and the emotional effects on the recipients are the same as if the abuse was intentional.

Natural to be emotionally affected

Even for the most knowledgeable and experienced partners and family members, it is still impossible to adequately insulate oneself or undertake enough self-talk to prevent feeling hurt or emotionally affected in some way.   To become unaffected or numb would indicate the sad loss of some normal and healthy aspects of being emotionally "typical", and indicate a need for counselling or psychological support to restore emotional health.

Incidents in common

So, why does abuse seem to be a common feature in the marriage and family relationships that we are aware of?

A look at the features of Asperger's Syndrome leads one to the conclusion that relationships are going to be impacted on significantly. Asperger's Syndrome involves difficulties with many aspects of communication, as well as social instinct, attention, planning, prioritizing, organizing, self-insight, emotion and sensory management, etc.

Common descriptions of behaviours reported by partners and family members do include verbal aggression, blame, disproportionate emotional reactions, frequent criticism and correction, withdrawal, retaliation, etc. Time and time again we hear comments on how "angry" the person with Asperger's Syndrome seems most of the time, and yet in most instances the person with Asperger's Syndrome will deny that they are angry.

Contradicting perceptions of incidents seem to be a common occurrence and these result in an enormous amount of conflict, often leading to destructive "tit for tat" exchanges and the build-up of mistrust, both ways.

Problems with self-insight, discernment and appropriateness

Once one has knowledge and understanding of Asperger's Syndrome, the reasons why these behaviours take place makes sense. Typically an individual with Asperger's Syndrome does not seem to have insight or awareness to help them discern whether or not their tone, effect or words are appropriate for a particular situation, and will be resistant to receiving feedback, often taking great offence when the partner or family member attempts to discuss or negotiate these types of incidents. In parenting situations this can leave a parent unable to protect a child from mistreatment by an Asperger parent, because agreement cannot be reached on the definition or existence of the alleged abusive attitude or behaviour.

Disability or disorder that can't be helped or a difference that can be managed?

So, herein lies the dilemma, do we re-define the meaning of abuse just because a person has Asperger's Syndrome and lacks awareness or insight into how their behaviours are being experienced by the significant others in their lives?

I suspect that to do this just reinforces the concept that Asperger's Syndrome is a disorder or disability that can't be helped rather than a difference that can be accepted, embraced and managed.

However, to accept, embrace and manage one's "difference" requires an openness and willingness on the part of the person with Asperger's Syndrome to acknowledge his or her own areas of difficulty and weakness, much the same as a "typical" person must be open and willing to acknowledge personality and character weaknesses if they want to grow in maturity as an adult and positively nurture their relationships.

Denial reinforces abuse

What makes our experiences so much more painful is the common response by people with Asperger's Syndrome to resist or deny any suggestion that they possess Asperger characteristics or are behaving in the ways we are attempting to describe to them. This resistance and denial reinforces many times over the impact of any abuse, and renders partners and family members powerless to effect positive change or growth in the relationship, or effect accountability in any way.

Whilst there are countless adults with Asperger's Syndrome who have accepted and embraced their Asperger "difference", the testimonies of partners who continue to seek support from partner support groups such as ASPIA, indicate that there are still countless married men and women with significant Asperger characteristics who have not explored or accepted their own difficulties or weaknesses and are therefore not embracing or managing them. Consequently this increases and compounds the burden that non-Asperger partners and family members experience in relation to the unequal sharing of responsibility within marital and family relationships, and leaves them powerless to protect themselves from ongoing abuse, opposition or deprivation within the home.

Non-Asperger partners can behave abusively too

It is also important to state at this point that without an adequate understanding and embracing of Asperger's Syndrome by both partners in a relationship, the risk of mutual abuse is very high. Non-Asperger partners and family members do resort to abusive attitudes and behaviours within relationships and family contexts too. It is essential that partners and family members seek support and professional guidance to help them cope with the confusing complexities and frustrations that occur in a relationship where Asperger's Syndrome is being poorly managed or not managed at all.

Dignity and respect for all

No-one would deny the right of people with Asperger's Syndrome to be accepted and treated with equal respect and dignity as any other human being on this earth, but the appeal goes forth from partners and partner groups like ours to those adults who are demonstrating Asperger characteristics to please explore, accept, embrace and responsibly manage their behaviours in the same way that every adult on this earth is expected to in order to avoid abusive expressions and behaviours towards the partners, children, family members and friends who care for them the most and who are deserving of the same respect and dignity.

In writing this article I do personally feel emotionally pulled in two opposing directions.

One is the desire to be merciful towards those individuals with Asperger's Syndrome known to me who I know are doing the best they can in their own particular circumstances.

The other pull I feel is the reason why I have gone ahead and written this article, which is my awareness and concern for thousands of situations where partners, children and family members remain powerless and voiceless within homes where an undiagnosed or resistant adult with the traits of Asperger's Syndrome persists unchecked in perpetrating acts of bullying or abuse towards partners and family members.

These behaviours are often carried out in order to maintain control over the home and family environment, ensure predictability and a prescribed order, preserve their own status or pride or sustain the screen of self-protection they hide behind to avoid confronting their own issues of anxiety, depression, anger, fear and pain.

It is my hope that adults with Asperger's Syndrome everywhere will seek information and professional help for the sake of their own well-being, and also for the sake of the family members who share life and home with them.

Carol Grigg© 2012

Essay – Change takes Time

As the co-ordinator of a support group for partners of adults with Asperger's Syndrome, most of the phone calls and emails I receive are from partners who have just discovered that Asperger's Syndrome could be what is affecting their situation.

Their search had become one of desperation as their emotional and physical reserves are near depletion and they are losing hope for the relationship, and in some cases, the whole family.

The discovery of Asperger's Syndrome can be an exciting relief, bringing renewed hope and some renewed energy … for a while … until we realise that there is no magic wand.

This part of the journey can be very dark, and it is usual to feel like everything we ever knew has been tossed upside-down and we don't know which way is upright anymore. The discovery of Asperger's Syndrome requires that we re-think the way we view everything and the way we approach everything within our relationship and family. On top of the immense effort that has already been channelled into surviving the situation and searching for an answer, this can seem beyond overwhelming.

It is at this point we need to be merciful towards ourselves and allow for a process to take place over time.

With the search over, it is important to take time to learn more about Asperger's Syndrome and understand where the behaviours are coming from. Time gives you an opportunity to seek professional help for information and guidance. Time provides an opportunity for you to experience the validation that a peer support group like ASPIA can provide. Time will allow you to begin the process of healing and recovery for yourself. Time gives you a chance to think everything through carefully before you make an attempt to introduce the possibility of AS to your partner, family or friends if and when the time is finally right. Time gives you an opportunity to reflect and to forgive yourself, releasing all the guilt you feel from not knowing and understanding it was a disorder. You did the best you could with what you knew.

With time you will find you can let your partner off the hook for some things, and you will develop the wisdom you need in order to know what behaviours and characteristics are harmful to yourself and the family and that need addressing.

For the partners who've acknowledged they may have Asperger's Syndrome, change will still take time, sometimes a long time. People with AS have difficulty with change and adaptability at the best of times, so presenting to them that they've got it "wrong" could be enough to cause a shut down or a melt-down, and could explain a lot of the denial and hostility we experience from them.

Professional guidance and supervision of this process is seriously recommended. An adult with Asperger's Syndrome won't know how or what to change. They won't have a Plan B or an alternative way of doing daily life. Some non-AS partners have observed that as they themselves calmed down and began to quietly change their own expectations and behaviours, their partners with AS began to move towards them and develop curiosity about what was going on. This is the kind of opportunity we all pray for – let's keep praying!

Carol Grigg

Section 3 A Wealth of Helpful Information

Quick Tips

Essential things to remember every day …

- People with Asperger's Syndrome are typically highly anxious, but may not recognize their anxiety.
- They may be experiencing feelings, but not be able to recognize which feelings they are or how to express them appropriately.
- It is important for partners to reduce the emotional atmosphere in the home and the relationship as much as possible.
- When an Asperger person senses that we're getting emotional they may withdraw or retreat, or escalate.
- They may escalate in order to shut us down or get us to back off, sometimes simply because they don't feel they can keep up with the verbal exchange with us.
- Being controlling can be about reducing anxiety and unpredictability.
- We cannot out-escalate them, so don't try. Just back away from the exchange or call for time out.
- It may be necessary for them to reach meltdown level in order to soothe themselves and calm down again, like a pressure release valve.
- Stress may strengthen the Asperger traits.
- They may be controlling in order to prevent situations happening where they don't know what to do.
- May cope better when there is more order and predictability.
- As stress increases, tolerance for the sensations of physical affection and intimacy may reduce.
- May have difficulty with more than one role at once such as being a partner and a parent.
- Have trouble shifting attention from one task or activity to another.
- May need time and space to calm down and shift attention after coming home from work. Avoid demands at this time.
- Try to avoid unexpected changes or surprises. Plan and give information ahead of time.
- They have trouble processing verbal communication on the spot – words, meaning, gist, and when combined with body language, facial expression, tone and emotion, communication can go haywire every time, and very quickly.
- Must say what we mean and not rely on them to pick up on implied meaning, or to interpret what we're meaning.
- They may become overwhelmed by commotion, too many people, public places, noisy environments and background hums.
- They may become overloaded by too many social engagements.
- Need to allow time and space for them to calm down and re-group between social events, relationship encounters or work demands.
- Special interests can help them calm down and become soothed, so can work in favour of the relationship if they are contained.

- They tend to approach every situation as though it's a new and different situation, and don't generalize what they know from one situation to another.
- May not initiate or reciprocate and may need to be prompted frequently to do things.
- May respond well to lists of tasks or notes on a planner.
- Try using email to communicate. This eliminates all the hazards of face-to-face communication and allows them time to understand the meaning and think before responding.
- They don't perceive when their tone and manner are inappropriate and impacting negatively on other people. Try not to take this personally.
- Be merciful to yourself too. Partners are human and have limitations as well. Ensure you have adequate time to be who you are and do things you enjoy or find restorative.
- A relationship is only safe if you know you can leave if you want to.
- A major contributor to depression in women is a lack of options or choices.

Essential Tips for getting through Conflict

- Keep the emotional atmosphere calm.
- Be curious rather than critical.
- Keep your words simple, direct and logical.
- Clarify meaning.
- Avoid ambiguity.
- One person speaking at a time.
- Be aware of anxiety building up, turn your body/eyes away. If already stressed, back off immediately.
- Limit or narrow your requests and responses (rather than expanding or elaborating, ie, don't bring in more and more arguments and reasons).
- Stick with the current issue and keep it simple.
- Avoid being confrontational.
- If anxiety rises for either, suggest a time-out and then try again a bit later.
- Using email has the benefit of eliminating emotion and allowing them time to think before they respond.

ASPIA's Self-Care Suggestions

Collection of Ideas by ASPIA group members 6 June 2009

Caring for ourselves . . .

- Put "self" on the agenda
- It's ok to be who I am, like what I like, do things I enjoy; I don't have to only do what my partner approves of
- Create own little space, a desk, use earphones, place of refuge
- Ok to have time for myself
- Do separate activities from partner
- Watch own TV shows, enjoy comedy, laugh
- Find own identity, protect own time
- Have some quiet time
- Ok to have a holiday separate from partner
- Eat properly
- Walk, swim, jog, exercise, massage, yoga, dancing, dancing lessons
- Do classes or a course – art, music, etc
- Have independent income, employment
- Pre-organise support from friends or family following surgery
- Enjoy pets
- Help others
- Spiritual dimension – faith, prayer
- Receive personal counselling
- Release thoughts and feelings by writing in a journal
- Get own anxieties under control (partner may mirror my anxieties)
- Don't get trapped into feeling like you need to justify your needs or existence

Remembering our need for friends . . .

- Get rid of negative friends and choose positive friendships
- Re-establish social times – coffee, movie, etc with friends
- Join a singing group or choir
- Holiday with a friend
- Walk with friends
- Manage phone plans to be able to afford keeping good contact with friends and family
- Attend a support group
- Allow other people in, don't withdraw or isolate

Coping better as a partner . . .

- Understand Asperger's Syndrome and the Asperger "landscape"
- Step back from emotional situations
- Let some things go
- Go around things, not through
- Separate living quarters may help
- Actual separation
- Have options – "If you feel you can leave, then the relationship is safe."
- Adjust your expectations of partner, self and relationship
- Separate Asperger's Syndrome from the person

- Explore partner's perception of me – am I perceived by him/her as being aggressive?
- Remember that people with AS hate conflict
- Learning, thinking, change own mind-set to see problem as opportunity to learn
- Stop seeing self as victim; see self as active member of the relationship
- Emotionally screen out negative words/actions, allow yourself to receive positive words/actions
- Love & commitment – there is a bond, in spite of it all
- Find the right distance between myself and partner that enables me to respect him/her
- Sow seeds of suggestion, allow time
- Give time for AS partner to process things – maybe days or even longer
- Allow them some space
- Allow them some time for their interests
- Realise they understand intellectually not emotionally
- Have flexible plans – build in space and time around plans
- Plan around the reality

Understanding does make a Difference: Insights and Suggestions for Caring for Ourselves

Many of these suggestions come directly from partners themselves, and also professional presentations at ASPIA meetings

Information and Insights

- By always deferring to our partners' needs, we actually end up with less time to grow and develop ourselves as people.
- We probably need more help and support for ourselves than we realize.
- We have a lot of love to give, but our Asperger partner won't recognize what we're giving at the level we would recognize if that love was being given to us.
- It is very hard for the non-Asperger partner to have their neurotypical needs met in an AS/NT relationship or to feel a sense of satisfaction within it (this can also be true of any relationship).
- We may struggle in our parenting role because we did not anticipate the unequal sharing of parenting responsibilities that eventuates.
- We are victims of our own need for expression of love. We extend self, but receive little or nothing back.
- We cannot exist in an emotional vacuum.
- Those who have a big heart in a relationship or family where that is not ok will get hurt. Will be made to feel like the odd one out and that we're not ok.
- We (NT partners) have different expectations and beliefs about change, but most of us have a lot more capacity to change than we realize.
- If I change, it may open up possibilities of my AS partner changing.
- Our own childhood experiences set up meaning for us about what's going on in our lives now. We may tolerate a lot more because it feels normal, and it fits our view of what to expect. Cultural and religious background may set people up to tolerate a lot more.
- If I become more and more responsible, partner may become more and more dependent. We can create a rod for our own backs. Just because I may choose to become less responsible doesn't mean that they'll then become more responsible. More than likely they will continue in the pattern that has been established over time.
- We all have a tendency to base how we feel about ourselves on someone else, and lack a concept of our real self.
- When we're unwell or struggling emotionally we can become delusional.
- We all have beliefs and rules about how things are supposed to be done.
- We have the ability to meet other people on a whole range of different levels.
- We have some similar characteristics to our partners, and some modeling takes place.
- Safety is paramount in the relationship; it may harm me to stay.
- Remember that it is not only the AS partner who is capable of abuse within the relationship.
- What is keeping me in this relationship? Is my safety radar not working? There may be lots of reasons for staying, but some may be my own dependence.
- To safely stay in the relationship, I have to be able to leave. Have to be able to make a choice.
- We often lack emotional support from family members and friends because they do not understand or appreciate the extra, "hidden" strains placed on a relationship by Asperger's Syndrome.

- We can end up dangerously isolated.
- It is common to have doubts about the integrity of the relationship and wonder whether or not we should end it.
- Problems in the relationship do not seem to improve despite great effort on our part.
- We find it difficult to understand or accept that our partner will not recover from Asperger's Syndrome or become "typical", and this can provoke feelings of guilt, despair and disappointment.
- Neurotypicals tend to only notice information that has social relevance.
- My partner will pick up on my anxiety and stress levels and may mirror them.

Suggestions and Strategies

- Give yourself plenty of time out.
- Pursue information and support for own sake
- Adjust personal expectations and attitudes
- Don't take anything personally.
- Use anti-depressants or anti-anxiety medication if your own anxiety is getting too high and preventing you from self-soothing.
- Have an exercise routine. This is great for self-soothing and feeling better and also for having some time out from the home situation.
- Focus on what you need to do for yourself and follow through for your own sense of fulfilment or accomplishment.
- Reserve time and energy for self-growth.
- Partner must get some or all of our neurotypical needs met outside of the relationship.
- I must recognize my strong needs for love and affection and do something about it. The worst thing I can do for myself is to ignore this need.
- Must accept the reality of the situation and settle, or pull the plug and get out.
- Learn how to manage stress and burn-out.
- Give out, but be realistic about what I expect back, because it won't always be what I want. It will be up to me to adjust and adapt myself and my expectations.
- Learn how to adjust my expectations (in general within the home) so that I don't wear out. May have to be happy with things being less than what I want in order to avoid burning out or disappearing entirely.
- I have to take responsibility for me.
- Learn to facilitate, not caretake.
- Check with myself regularly about how I'm going about having my emotional and intimacy needs met.
- It is important for us to grow. We need to take the time to unpack our own issues and seek help for sorting them out.
- How real are my perceptions? Get someone else to help me sort this out.
- Be aware of my own limitations and boundaries.
- If I set up rules I may not be able to change this later. Need to yield a little now to avoid burn-out down the track.
- Necessary to get used to solitude.
- Need more self-care.
- Don't fuse and merge into partner. Keep integrity of who I am – the good, the bad and the ugly.
- Keep sense of self, and grow.

- Figure out where I am, and where I need to go to.
- We have choices in life. It may not feel like we do, but we may just be unaware of the choices we have.
- Gratitude will help my attitude.
- It has been suggested that I verbalise my thinking when the AS person is around so that they know my process.

Understanding does make a Difference: Insights and Suggestions specific to the Relationship

Many of these ideas have come directly from group members and others come from professional presentations at ASPIA meetings

Information and Insights

- The only people who can learn are those who want to learn.
- There are a whole set of gestures and language that don't take place in a relationship where Asperger's Syndrome is present.
- We tend to assume that they "get" what we "get".
- The traditional husband role is as "provider". Difficult for any husband to accept when he can't meet his wife's emotional needs. This can be an intolerable thought, and could be difficult for an Asperger husband to live with.
- An Asperger partner may become more Asperger as they get older.
- Most of us, either Neurotypical or Asperger, are operating at the lowest level of change possibility.
- Relationships are a dance between two people and we have developed patterns of dancing in our relationship. We may have developed bad habits, and may have set up co-dependence.
- What often makes a difference to us is what meaning we give to the behaviours of our partner, and vice versa. This is influenced by how we see life and what our own experiences have been in our family of origin and in other relationships.
- When a relationship is under stress, people go into survival mode. They become linear and their IQ drops.
- Stress and fatigue are killers for all of us.
- Remember that when we and our partners come home at the end of the day we are weary and spent. Unfortunately this means that we are interacting when we are at our worst and we both give and get the dregs.
- Our partners will shut down if an experience becomes too intense.
- If our partners pick up emotional intensity they will see it as a threat. They will either come out fighting or go into a hole.
- It takes a lot of time for our Asperger partners to ease the nervous energy out of their system.
- We get angry and resentful, partner responds by shutting down. We do help to set up problems.
- Trauma causes rigidity for anyone. Emotion can send an AS person into a post-traumatic stress reaction. There's a lot of trauma going both ways in the relationship. It may be for different reasons, but it is happening. Both partners could have a previous history of trauma.
- Some partners have noticed that there seems to be a cycle taking place, ie, improvement for a while following a crisis or breakthrough, then a slow deterioration again.
- Remember that an AS parent and AS child may have very different sensory needs, so forcing family togetherness or joint activities may create a disaster.
- Remember that change will take time.

- The advice and strategies provided by counsellors that promote togetherness do not work in these relationships. More separateness may actually help improve the relationship.
- Can't out-escalate an Asperger person. They can keep escalating and won't pull themselves back. They want to pursue their "truth" to the end as it makes so much sense to them. They feel like they lose all the time, so they will keep going.
- If either partner won't or can't learn, very little progress can be made.
- Asperger partner may be less sexually active than we expect because they know it comes with their partner's need for emotional connection.
- On the other hand, sex could end up being an obsessive interest with some Asperger adults.
- Being married and having children could be a status thing socially.
- May not read situations properly with children, particularly intent or the "what ifs". Safety could be an issue. May freeze in new situations with a child in their care.
- We never know what to expect because we're not aware of what's been happening for them prior to the present context. They seem to have more fluctuations than the average person. When they're struggling there will be more trouble. When they (or us) lose it, the IQ drops.
- When the whole system is calm, frontal lobes (wisdom) are in control. When we are stressed, aroused, depressed we have less frontal lobe in control and more limbic (survival) system in control, this equals tunnel vision, the big picture is reduced, common sense goes, ability to handle emotional situations reduced, cognitive ability changes.
- Our verbal ability is threatening to them.
- Their expressive ability (inability) may be perceived by us as withdrawal, but they actually can't articulate.
- Lots of AS partners had parents with Aspergers, and will have experienced a faulty attachment process.
- We can contribute to setting up problems.
- If I become more and more responsible, partner may become more and more dependent. We can create a rod for our own backs. Just because I may choose to become less responsible doesn't mean that they'll then become more responsible. More than likely they will continue in the pattern that has been established over time.
- Some relationships are abusive, and it is not just the AS partner that abuses.
- Safety is paramount, for either partner. Both partners can have inappropriate responses. It may harm us to stay.
- We are de-masculinising our male AS partners if we only criticize.
- Tension in the relationship will strengthen the AS traits in our partner.
- Our AS partners may show their love for us by what they do for us.

Suggestions and Strategies

- Suggest professional consultation, give "helping the relationship" or "improving understanding" as the reason.
- If a specific change is desired or necessary for the well-being of the relationship or family, giving an ultimatum may work, but only after careful consideration and planning, and preferably seeking professional guidance and support.
- When communicating, keep to one topic at a time.
- When initiating a discussion, lead in with preparatory words as an introduction, maybe request a specific time, place and time-frame for the discussion (ie 15 mins).
- Try using email to discuss issues, or to request a time for discussion.

- Stick to agreed plan or topic.
- Maybe go out for dinner to talk (being in a public place can prevent escalation).
- Talk in the dark (less confronting, removes body language, eye contact)
- Use a whiteboard for discussions, write things down, summarise & even leave things written up as a reminder.
- Use a calendar or planner. This has helped marvelously in some situations. Remember that AS people are usually visual – need a visual prompt that is clear, simple and where they will see it.
- Give specific times for certain activities, etc.
- Avoid surprises as much as possible, give time for AS person to prepare.
- Keep a journal of what has been agreed or the results of a discussion.
- Only spend time together when it will be positive, like going out for dinner, etc.
- When AS partner gets home from work, give him space for at least 15 minutes (some need longer) before you even speak to him, and especially before you make requests or generally try to engage with him.
- Give AS person a transition time from one situation to another (work to home, social situations, etc). Need time to disengage and unwind.
- Be prepared to change some routines in the home.
- Maybe stagger the times you leave for work or arrive home from work, so you both don't leave or arrive at the same time.
- Don't assume anything.
- Pause, don't react.
- When you take a stand, do it calmly & firmly, and don't back down.
- When you take a stand, be prepared for World War III or a meltdown. This seems to be normal, but often passes if you hold your ground calmly and don't react or allow yourself to escalate or be intimidated.
- Be prepared to follow through if you make a threat, and make the choice of outcome theirs.
- Be happy in the silence, side by side is ok.
- Ask them specifically "What do you want from me?"
- Clearly define what you want from them. Give clear instructions. Keep it simple.
- Avoid using a controlling tone of voice, be as neutral as possible and preferably negotiate by email so emotion is eliminated and AS partner has time to think.
- Do deals with them, exchange requests.
- Acknowledge any improvements and express how it makes you feel better.
- May work well to divide the house so AS partner has a separate area all of his own. Can still share responsibilities and a love-life, but the rest of the time is spent separately.
- Family dinners together can be a disaster.
- Ensure you have the support of an experienced counsellor or psychologist if you're taking a stand at home. Support is essential.
- Detach lovingly by excusing yourself from the interaction when you feel it is escalating or becoming stressful.
- Respect their need for a space of their own to retire to when stressed.
- Sow seeds of suggestion calmly & firmly, but don't be in their face, quietly wait.
- Try to avoid conveying that they are defective.
- One partner calmly stated to her AS husband that she was going to take a holiday by herself each year. Initially her husband was resistant, but now accepts this. She enjoys planning for it and organizes the family for while she's away. Looking forward to this helps her to cope better throughout the year.

- One partner presented to her AS husband in a calm and logical manner that she had noticed she seemed to be the cause of his anger. She stated that the anger had to stop, and so therefore she must leave the relationship so that the anger can stop. Her husband responded positively and change has begun for them.
- One partner calmly threatened a marital separation unless her conditions were met. He didn't take her seriously and failed to meet the conditions, so she left just as she had warned. He responded by co-operating with her conditions.
- One partner calmly informed her husband that she was going to return to University to gain a further qualification. Her husband was resistant, but she followed through and he accepted it.
- We must stop trying to make our Asperger partner neurotypical.
- Seek to find a common understanding of what keeps you together; what's important to both of you.
- Need to find a "currency" that works for me – is my reaction extreme or obvious enough to have an impact?
- A logical argument will always work better than strongly expressed emotions.
- Can the Asperger partner see that a change will be beneficial for him/her?
- If I change, it may open up possibilities of my AS partner changing.
- Try not to be a sabre tooth tiger – we can be one of their stressors. If they perceive us as threatening then that is their reality.
- We can tone things down, and we need to learn to do this.
- We need to have realistic expectations and perceptions. What meaning do we put on these expectations and perceptions? Make sure our perceptions are accurate.
- To be successful in the relationship we need to be flexible and realistic. Know where reality is and work with that reality.
- Work as a couple to make it work. I have to take responsibility for me. The more we work with reality, the more successful we'll be.
- If we do something that doesn't work, it will come back and hit us in the face.
- Work within their reality too.
- Help facilitate without taking responsibility. Facilitate, not caretake. Allow them their dignity.
- When communicating, use logic with no (or less) emotion. Make it short and concise, more analytical and logical. As soon as emotion is introduced they're gone. They can't follow us once emotion is introduced.
- Communicate in an intellectual, calm way so they don't feel threatened.
- Attend, empathise, be intellectual.
- Use lay terms about relationship difficulties rather than naming AS.
- If AS partner is comfortable, ask for input and perspective from someone else who is trusted, may help to show up differences.
- We can have some of our needs met with our partners because there are some similarities between us (drawn together initially). Need to re-discover these and find a way to enjoy them together again.
- Intimacy can be intellectual, physical or emotional. Physical can include watching a movie, etc, side-by-side "play". Think beyond the obvious for ideas.
- Work place stays mostly intellectual. Create a "working relationship" with partner.
- A reward can be the enjoyment of intellectual conversations together.
- We must affirm them and reflect positives.

Understanding does make a Difference: Insights and Suggestions for understanding People with Asperger's Syndrome

Most of the following information has been gleaned from professional presentations at ASPIA meetings or workshops

Information and Insights

- May have trouble choosing words or formulating a question.
- May need external prompts
- Lack simultaneous sense of self and other, particularly when social interaction is initiated by other.
- Have trouble shifting attention from one thing to another
- Written or visual information is more easily assimilated
- May stay with a topic that is familiar to them or safe
- May have only one blueprint that is used for all situations
- May be fearful of the following:
- Direct confrontation
- Too many people talking at once
- Highly stimulating, busy or noisy environments
- Waiting in queues
- Discussions that move into emotions (eg, how do you think I feel?)
- Focus being on him/her, rather than an event
- Making mistakes
- Why questions. Asking him/her to explain his/herself or his/her actions is difficult because it is particularly difficult to back-track.
- Are generally highly anxious
- Hoarding may be related to:
  - Fear
  - Anxiety
  - Loss of control
  - Concern with error
  - Predictability and future order
  - Indecision
  - Disorganisation
  - Perfectionism
  - Procrastination
  - Internal chaos (etc)
- Routine & repetition lowers arousal and reduces mental energy (lessens processing load)
- May be pre-occupied with retaining sameness at the expense of difference or change
- Simpler for them to see things as black & white, good or bad, right or wrong, rather than looking at complexity
- Behaviours like staring, delayed response, irrelevant response, restlessness, leaving the scene, aggression, may just be a cover for the internal labour involved in translating and processing information.
- Delayed processing may result in gaps in important and relevant information, preventing them from completing a concept or task.

- Are typically happy when they please their partner, unhappy when they don't, BUT, they do not know why their partner is happy or unhappy. To them, it either happens or not. They cannot generalize and repeat it for another time.
- Respond best to experience, not theory or value systems.
- Cannot understand implied meaning or references in either literature or personal communication.
- Behaviours like word wars, repetitive questions, not waiting for answers, oppositional behaviours, abuse, etc may be related to a fear of not understanding.
- May not recognize their own signs of anxiety or be able to self-soothe.
- May need to have a meltdown in order to defuse stress, self-soothe and re-compose themselves.
- May project their emotions and provoke us, which in effect takes the focus off them.
- May not initiate relationship exchanges.
- May need prompting.
- May automatically be resistant to change of any kind.
- Anxiety develops from cumulative effect of missing bits of conversation and what's going on.
- Talking non-stop may be a way of preventing reciprocal interaction.
- Asperger person wants to control their environment in order to reduce their own anxiety, and we just happen to be in it.
- They can tend to pay back what they perceive we are doing or saying to them, tit for tat, eg, if we tell them they're controlling they will look for situations where they perceive we are being controlling and will criticize us for that.
- For them, trust is based on facts, actions, behaviours. For us, we rely on instinct to know who we can trust.
- For an Asperger person absense of conflict equals a Neurotypical's state of "happiness" and is a favourable state.
- They may believe that their mood changes are caused by external sources, including other people.
- They may go to lengths to ensure we won't ask anything of them or impose on them.
- They may not get the meaning of something until it happens to them.
- They have difficulty expressing emotions in words. They may not be able to find the words because the emotion's meaning is unknown and lost to them.
- Their learning is situation-specific. May see someone crying but not relate it to himself until it happens to him.
- An Asperger person's moral compass may be provided by the church.
- They are rule-based thinkers.
- They hear "I'm wrong ..." over and over again, and attack back.
- They know that something's going on but have no idea what. This leads to anxiety.
- Some people with AS will only notice extreme emotion, and they do care.
- Some people with AS won't notice emotion in others, and/or don't care.
- Although empathy is lacking, compassion may well be very present but "mistimed".
- Remember that Asperger's Syndrome in the population is still a new and emerging field. There are many variations and differences, and many are still being missed.
- Variations in ability may not be "very" different, just a "bit more of" or a "bit less of".
- Remember it is a systemic difference, not just neurology.
- They have a limited capacity for change. It can be depressing thinking that the AS won't move or shift, but most people with AS can change, just in a limited way. Some are stuck and can't change at all, but this is a small minority.

- Emotional maturity stops around puberty. When stress increases they go back to puberty.
- Lots of AS partners had parents with Aspergers, and will have experienced a faulty attachment process.
- People with AS have more ups and downs. When there's more movement internally, mood related delusions can occur.
- They will miss the subtle messages that are conveyed by facial expressions, eye contact and body language.
- When people lack an understanding of Asperger's Syndrome, they will make a moral judgment about the person with AS and their behaviours.
- AS person looks for certainty.
- Brain has trouble amplifying one voice and drowning out background noise.
- Have trouble converting thought and emotion into speech.
- Solve social problems using their intellect, and brain works hard.
- Tend to notice errors and spot differences, not similarities.
- They are distracted from within.
- They feel defective and depressed.
- Arrogance may be a compensation for not fitting in.
- Desperation for acceptance could come across as gender confusion.
- Tend to escape into their own world.
- Major organization problems (executive function) may emerge in puberty.
- Easily distracted, lose train of thought, have to start again.
- If they can't make something work, they won't know to try another way and will keep trying. Don't have flexibility in thinking.
- See detail but miss the overall picture, pattern or gist (themes).
- Can't determine what's relevant and what's redundant, have different priorities.
- Overwhelmed in new situations.
- They look for or try to create a pattern or order, or they panic. Life is chaotic.
- Constant change prevents preparation.
- Fear of making a mistake may lead to them not trying.
- May be perfectionistic.
- Have a limited frustration for tolerance.
- Special interests keep them calm. Be realistic and merciful about allowing and managing these.
- Will pick up on anxieties and stress levels of those around them, including partner and family members.
- They are surprisingly sensitive to the personality of a teacher, or other adult.
- They have an instinct for who likes them and who doesn't.
- An AS teacher (or parent) may be the least likely to understand a child with AS.
- Emotion and chaos leads to disintegration.
- They can't inhibit their sensory experiences.
- They don't perceive, prioritise or process the social world.
- They may express in music or through movies or pets, etc, rather than with words.
- Have trouble reading own thoughts and feelings - self-reflection.
- Have trouble reading the thoughts and feelings of others – theory of mind.
- Degree of stress is proportionate to number of people present.
- They repair either by destruction, solitude or by blocking thoughts.
- Won't identify their own negative emotion until they're beyond managing it.
- May be over sensitive to external danger, but unaware of imminent internal meltdown.

- May misinterpret people's reactions, look at the act not the intention.
- They may associate laughter with ridicule because of past experiences.
- May make incorrect assumptions.
- Alcohol and marijuana are relaxants, but these cause emotional and intellectual maturity to freeze.
- One in four people with AS will have Obsessive Compulsive Disorder (OCD).
- Many will have Post-Traumatic Stress Disorder (PTSD) which may come from experiencing bullying.
- They may ruminate over errors, and anxiety about the next day.
- May be controlling or avoidant.
- They can learn dysfunctional strategies in order to control a situation or escape, eg, blackmail, manipulation, etc.
- Special interests can be a way of managing behaviours.
- Depression is very common.
- Most are very aware of being different, and have low self-esteem due to being rejected and ridiculed.
- May be lonely and be experiencing mental exhaustion.
- May have depression attacks, much like panic attacks.
- Some attempt suicide.
- Two out of three people with AS have anger management problems.
- Anger can be an expression of sadness and anxiety.
- They may externalize anger and direct blame at others.
- Anger management problems may actually be clinical depression.
- They may either become clinically depressed, or go on the attack.
- Features of AS may fluctuate and be variable from day to day.
- They don't like "no", "wait".
- They don't like change, frustration, sensory overload, unfamiliar or confusing circumstances, shouting.
- They can't explain what happened – they will experience more agitation if they are put under pressure.
- There may be a family history of mood disorder.
- They can tend to catastrophise.
- Emotions confuse their thinking.
- Special interest can help with overcoming fear, keeping anxiety under control, blocking angry or anxious thoughts, and as a means of relaxation and pleasure.
- An angry reaction could mean high anxiety, or clinical depression.
- Girls with Aspergers tend to be philosophers and boys tend to be professors.
- If religious, they tend towards the God of Retribution in the Old Testament rather than Jesus Christ of forgiveness in the New Testament.
- Special interest can be a search for a simpler or happier world.

Suggestions and Strategies

- Keep the emotional atmosphere calm
- Be curious rather than critical
- Explain things carefully with enough detail
- Put as much information as possible in visual form and leave it around the house, eg, diagrams, photos, timetables, written messages; include who; what; when; where; why;
- Allow extra time for information to sink in (latent processing)
- Clear up misunderstandings/misperceptions as they arise

- Use straightforward, simple and logical language
- Be explicit and don't leave ambiguity
- One person at a time to speak
- Always prepare for change well in advance if possible
- Express routines in order of action
- Stick to routines
- Start sentences with what needs to be done, eg, "We need to get in the car at 10.30." rather than "If you don't get off the computer now, we'll never get to the shops."
- Show the beginning and end of a goal, then the steps on how to achieve the goal.
- Learn to recognize and be aware of signs of anxiety building up.
- Be alert to changes in them and respond appropriately.
- If confusion or anxiety arises, limit and narrow your requests and responses rather than expanding them or elaborating.
- Avoid confrontation.
- If they begin to become stressed, turn your body/eyes away.
- If already stressed, back off immediately.
- Social skills training is considered to be particularly helpful for the person with AS.
- Respect them for who they are and acknowledge their intellect.
- Teach them that calm = smart.
- Teach them that staying calm leads to quicker solutions.
- Teach them to ask for help.
- Teach them that mistakes are not a disaster, they are an opportunity to learn.
- Use logic, not punishment.
- Emotion management is important for social success.
- Best emotional restorative is solitude. It is important for home to be a safe haven.
- Learn relaxation therapies.
- May help them to keep a mood diary; use self-report scales; record of triggers.
- Important to reassure them that we are not angry with them.
- Provide compliments.
- Talk about things to look forward to.
- Need structure to organize emotional experiences.
- Need to be regularly taught about emotions, feelings, expression management.
- Knowledge about AS gives them the picture for the jigsaw puzzle.
- Ask permission to give them a hug.
- Find things that ease and release tension and plan these in.
- Use written explanations rather than verbal.
- Ensure a 1:1 ratio between socializing and solitude.
- Special interest can do what a "defrag" does for a computer.
- Special interest could be the "off" switch, may be only way to rescue a situation and calm down.
- Use logic to change behaviour. Becoming emotional adds fuel to fire.
- Don't remove special interest as a method of punishment.

Section 4 Newsletter "Thoughts": Validating and Supportive thoughts for the Journey

A Devastating Dearth of Information

In earlier Newsletters this year (2009) I have alluded to some controversies in the online forum communities of Asperger and Neurotypical people.

It has become necessary for us, as ASPIA, to recognise that we are no longer just a support group for partners and a website for information and contacts, but that our website is also seen by the wider communities as the representation of our group's attitudes towards those who are affected by Asperger's Syndrome.

The establishment of ASPIA was driven by a devastating dearth of information and support for those who, after many years and sometimes decades, "happened upon" the realisation that Asperger's Syndrome could be the unidentified factor creating unexplained confusion and frustration in their relationship, and influencing the steady and frightening erosion of what began as a solid and promising marriage.

Even if Asperger's Syndrome only affected communication between individuals in a relationship, communication in all its facets and complexities is the tool or key that enables us to successfully enter and share the world of another, mutually. This is what marriage is all about.

ASPIA has been dedicated to not only providing validation and support to non-Asperger partners, but to also providing education that enables growth of understanding.

Among many things, understanding will hopefully lead to improved communication between partners, and an easing of the confusion, frustration and erosion that has been taking place in these relationships.

The recent establishment of support groups for adults with Asperger's Syndrome is a promising new venture in the provision of education and support for individuals with AS who are in relationships.

Whilst we firmly believe that partners and families need information that clearly identifies and addresses the real issues in a relationship negatively affected by Asperger's Syndrome, we need to find balance in this. We recognise that to emphasise our own emotional damage in ways that personally denigrates our partners and places personal blame on them for all the relationship difficulties, we are inadvertently adding to further division in the relationship that will be counter-productive to what we really desire.

Upon discovery of AS, the tendency of the non-AS partner to blame the AS partner comes from a sense that they themselves have been shouldering an unfair load of blame for the relationship difficulties and it's hard not to want to point the finger back. When both partners come to an understanding of AS, the tendency to blame or retaliate diminishes.

ASPIA will continue to promote understanding, and believes that a supported partner can be the best ally an AS partner can have. However, ASPIA will also continue to emphasise that for couples, there is only so much influence that a supported partner can have within his or her relationship unless the partner with AS is also willing to participate in recognising the relationship difficulties being experienced and seeking mutually supportive solutions for the difficulties.

Our dream is that both partners can be mutual allies in re-building a relationship that works and creates emotional safety for both partners. Carol Grigg (October 2009)

A few words about loss and grief

We usually think of loss and grief in relation to someone passing away, a diagnosis of a life threatening disease or some significant life changing event involving the loss of something of great value to us.

For partners, the discovery of Asperger's Syndrome in our partner involves a whole range of feelings, which definitely include grief and a sense of loss. It's not a death, it's not a disease, and it's not a publicly recognisable loss. However, it is still a deep personal and private loss because all of our expectations, hopes and dreams suddenly have to change. Expectations of a normal, emotionally reciprocal relationship. Hopes that daily family life can be negotiated straightforwardly and provide healthy nurture and support for each family member. Dreams about normal future milestones including retirement, etc.

Many of these things can still be possible, but they will take a different form to what was naturally expected. The path forward will be altered and the steps will need to be more deliberate.

Feelings of loss and grief can seem like an engulfing fog, and may not be easily identified. It may help to talk to someone. I was greatly helped to work through a 10 week loss and grief programme* where I learned a lot about myself, my values and what was preventing me from healing and growing as an individual.

Being able to verbalise what the loss means to you will help you to gain greater objectivity about your pathway forward.

Carol Grigg, September 2008 (*Seasons for Growth, see www.goodgrief.org.au)

Jeroen Decates, Clinical Psychologist (Sydney), talking on "Hope & Despair", ASPIA meeting November 6, 2004 makes the following comment …

"Partners not only experience grief for the partner they didn't get, they experience grief for the partner they can't be … "

A Snapshot of Difficulties

One of the greatest things about attending our support group is the validation we each experience as we hear each other's stories and share our own. We recognise our own struggles in the struggles of others and realise we are not alone, which is very comforting. It also begins to ease away the feelings of isolation and aloneness that are a characteristic of each one of our lives, and reassures us that we are not crazy or imagining things.

In our last meeting (February 2012), we divided into smaller groups and, with the help of a printed hand-out, wrote down what we are finding the hardest to deal with at home at the moment.

I thought it could be beneficial to share some of these in this newsletter so that others on the mailing list can also experience the validation that those in the meeting did.

The things that group members were finding hard at the time of last month's meeting are as follows:

- Grief
- Perception of not having choices
- Not knowing where to place boundaries – what I will do and what I won't do
- Isolation, partner shutting down
- Disappointed expectations
- Unequal responsibility sharing
- Depression
- Lack of affection
- Anger
- Feelings of guilt
- Being blamed
- Control
- Change
- Clutter, disorganisation and hoarding
- Everything is just so hard, get stuck.

Perhaps more suggestions can be forwarded to us from others on the mailing list for inclusion on a group list for future discussions.

Carol, March 2012

A word of caution

Especially as the pressure of the Christmas season mounts.

If the frustration levels in your relationship have reached the point where either you or your partner are frequently resorting to acts of bullying or abuse towards each other, eg, shaming, humiliating, belittling in public, put-downs, yelling, criticism, needling, swearing, threatening, breaking or throwing things, physical harm, controlling, over-riding, intimidating, depriving, etc, then it is time to stop, think and make a decision about a temporary or permanent separation.

It is not ok to remain in & contribute to a relationship that is characterised by these behaviours, even if you hold Christian or traditional beliefs about marriage. Christian beliefs are primarily about love, kindness and self-control.

Harming a partner with attitudes, words or deeds is not ok for anyone, regardless of beliefs and regardless of one's neurology. No relationship can be recovered within that kind of atmosphere anyway.

"Time out" can work for adults too!

Carol Grigg (December 2011)

About Empathy

Empathy is "One person's attempt to experience the inner life of another while simultaneously retaining the stance of an objective observer." Heinz Kohut in Siegel & Hartzell (2005)

"There is always an emotional climate of respect and acceptance when there is empathy. This allows us to feel safe and free to reveal ourselves as we are, without the defensive barriers which we have erected over the years." (quoted from study material for Counselling course, AIPC).

Don't we all long to be in a family, group or community where this takes place, mutually?

I've been thinking a lot about empathy. So many things we read about Asperger's Syndrome state that people with AS do not have empathy. Some people with Asperger's Syndrome dispute this. I am wondering too.

Do they just appear to lack empathy because they are not reading the cues and non-verbal clues such as facial expression and body language? Some have suggested that they do have empathy but they just don't know how to express it. If they're uncertain about what is expected, perhaps it's safer not to risk getting it wrong. Some say they have so much empathy that it overwhelms and cripples them. Perhaps all of these possibilities are true. We know from testimonies that some people with AS are devastated when they finally realise how their actions or words have been hurting their partners. Sadly, others continue to combat every suggestion with denial, and some continue to remain absorbed only in what's happening for them.

Over the last two months I have been exchanging emails and thoughts with some adults with AS who accept & understand their own AS. I have been noticing that there is a significant flow of empathy in these exchanges that has surprised me and warmed my heart. It has occurred to me that, rather than being a barrier between partners, perhaps a computer screen could actually become a conductor to re-connect the hearts and minds of people who were once friends. In our meetings we mention that writing to or emailing our partners could assist with communication. It seems to be face to face situations that are too much for an AS person to process - the words, the tone, the volume, the facial expression, the body language, the emotion – all at once. Emailing eliminates most of these aspects and allows time for thought and response.

I know we long for meaningful face-to-face communication, but perhaps there are some things we have to accept in our journey to understand AS. Maybe emailing can provide a stepping stone to new possibilities. … Carol (July 2009)

Accepting the reality

The following comments should really be submitted to a forum where they can be discussed. Our experiences are wide are varied, and my perspective on living with an AS partner is only one perspective among many valid experiences and perspectives.

I'll share my thoughts anyway: Some time back I found myself telling one of our members that she had to stop expecting her partner to suddenly become "normal" because in effect she was bashing her head against a brick wall, and this would only cause more harm to herself, and also the relationship.

I didn't mean this comment in any disrespectful way to either her or her partner. It's just a fact. Our partners have AS, and that's how it is. They will never become neurotypical, even though sometimes we may have the occasional "normal" interaction or situation that inspires hope that "normal" may be possible.

This led me to recognise how we naturally ache to find solutions in the context of our relationships. It's a natural bent or instinct within us. It is uncomfortable and unnatural to stay in that state of "un-solution", with no code or tool or key to hand that will bring "normal" and solutions. Incredibly disempowering actually. It's like living in a constant state of unfinished business, combined with confusion, day in and day out, and is probably quite a significant threat to our mental and emotional health, and our future outlook.

We just can't seem to get our heads around the fact that our AS loved one will remain AS and can't gradually make a transition to NT, in spite of now having answers and information. We naturally seem to have this expectation and assumption every day that something will finally fall into place or "click" and then from then on our discussions and communication will become "typical" and we'll understand and interpret each other accurately. It is so hard to live in this state of accepting this will never be; that AS is here to stay in the relationship dynamic; accepting that there will be no solution that will bring a sense of "normality"; no magic wand; no code breaker. I am sorry for the bleak outlook today but thank God we can now benefit from the "normalising" process of meeting and identifying with other partners."

Carol (June 2011)

Adapting to cope

When discussing AS partnerships recently with one of our partner-friends in Melbourne, I was reminded of how in our meetings we often note that our AS partners typically fall into one of two types or representations of expression, ie, aggressive/controlling and over-engaging, or passive/avoidant and detached. Like two extremes. It has also been observed in our meetings that non-AS partners often fall into one of two types of expression too.

It has been observed that many who attend group meetings are unusually lacking in confidence for their age, intelligence, life experience and vocation, and can seem quite down-trodden. Others are far more verbally and emotionally dominant, sometimes unusually aggressive and reactive.

It occurred to me that perhaps this could be related to how the non-AS partner's original personality type has changed or adapted to cope with the long-term effects of sharing life with a partner with one or the other type of AS expression, and are we seeing a corresponding extreme?

My personal experience was with a controlling, over-engaging AS partner and I was emotionally & verbally beaten down, powerless, imploding with grief and quiet rage and shattered in confidence. Perhaps those whose experience is with a passive/avoidant, detached type of AS partner may have become more aggressive and outwardly frustrated after years of trying to force engagement with an apparently unresponsive partner? Maybe I'm being overly simplistic, but always thinking …

I've mentioned before that the years of not knowing about AS, not understanding what was going on and not knowing how to respond constructively have done untold damage, no matter what our personality type. We've done our best at every point, and yet watched and felt our dreams, life-joy and sense of who we are crumbling away every day. This creates confusion, frustration, a sense of helplessness and a deep sense of loss.

For the sake of our emotional healing, we must remember how important it is to allow that ever-present bitterness to evolve into grief as we grow in our understanding of AS.

Carol (August 2011)

Being the Problem

During my time away on the North Coast a couple of weeks ago I spent a week with a dear old family friend. This friend and I have had many D & M's over the years, and we usually end up on the topic of her parents.

This friend has endured constant, inexplicable rejection and harassment from her parents, and sisters for her entire life. She is constantly agonizing over what she has done to deserve it … if only she could work it out and make amends … things could be resolved. But she hasn't a clue, and her parents just elude to things, and won't tell her what it is she's done wrong. The sense of guilt that plagues her has seriously affected her mental and emotional health, for many years now.

I was with this friend when she had one of those "aha" moments, when the pennies finally dropped and she realized that she is the problem, their problem … but not because she's done anything wrong. She is just her. And for some reason this has never been ok for her parents.

The burden that slipped off her shoulders was actually visible and measurable for me looking on. The guilt had been false guilt. Her steps became lighter, her voice stronger, her face came alive, the light and joy returned to her eyes, and she is still basking in this realisation. She's ok with being "the problem" because she's ok with who she is. Plenty of other people in her life love and respect her and value her for who she is.

That's not to say it isn't desperately painful to be rejected by those closest to us, but coming to a place of accepting and valuing ourselves for who we are, whether we're a problem to others or not, is a great milestone to reach.

I couldn't help thinking how this same realisation has helped many of us who have partners who seem to see us as "the problem" in their lives. The truth is, we are! But not because we've done anything wrong. We are simply being who we are. We have genuine needs for communication, affection, warmth, care, spontaneity – all "normal" needs for ordinary folk.

Let's be ok with being "the problem". It's surprisingly reassuring.

... Carol (February 2010)

"All persons should have the right to their own opinions and thoughts and should be in control of their own destiny, free to pursue their own interests in their own way as long as they do not trample on the rights of others." Carl Rogers.

Caught off-guard, again

I recently experienced a startling reminder of the unexpected and unpredictable difficulties that can occur when communicating with a loved one with Asperger tendencies.

This opening sentence in itself describes two of the most anxiety-producing aspects of communicating with someone with AS, namely:

1) that problems in communication happen when we're least expecting them, often over seemingly simple things or when things seem to be going along ok, and

2) that problems in communication happen unpredictably – sometimes they happen, sometimes they don't, they'll come from left-field and prevention seems so elusive.

What was highlighted in my recent experience was how difficult an AS person finds it to accept the validity of the meaning someone else places on a situation or experience when it is different to the meaning that same situation or experience has for them. In fact, the very existence of an opinion at variance to their own appears to represent a great dilemma for them, and even a threat to their emotional well-being.

I watched as panic set in in this dear one's eyes and demeanour. It was as though the very existence of a perspective different to their own meant to them that their own experience was entirely invalidated and that their personal rights and choices would be lost.

I felt cruel, yet all I wanted was to have my own perspective acknowledged as valid and equally worthy of existence alongside theirs.

What is so devastating and frustrating in relationships is that these episodes of "communication gone haywire" can end up being incredibly destructive to mutual trust and respect, and a residue of suspicion and mistrust begins to build up. It's particularly sad when this may just be due to a difference in the meaning each person ascribes to an experience.

When a place of mutual understanding and acceptance of differing perspectives cannot be reached, no compromise or agreement can be negotiated or resolution found and we are left with a breach or chasm that defies repair and de-stabilises the relationship at its deepest core. Sadly this is a dynamic that seems to be occurring frequently in AS/non-AS relationships, leading to a snowballing of unresolved issues over many years. Most couples need help and education to be able to untangle the gridlock that these experiences establish over time.

Thankfully in the situation I have described we had the benefit of understanding AS and were able to re-visit the matter when emotions had settled, talk objectively about the process that had taken place, recover our communication and build on the experience.

How I wish I'd had that sort of understanding 25 years ago. I know I'm not alone when I say "What a difference that could have made."

Carol (February, 2011)

Food for Thought

Our workshops with Tony Attwood & Isabelle Hènault (Sydney, March 2009) were riveting and amazing and so much was shared that would be impossible to convey adequately.

A few simple thoughts collected though are as follows . . .

It may be helpful to think more in terms of an "Asperger Personality Type".

The more the Asperger person feels confronted, the less the relationship is likely to work.

Know each other's limits socially – work out a strategy to limit our social expectations of our AS partners. Understand that they just don't cope.

The Asperger person's comfort zone may exclude their partner.

Future expectations

Many times in our support group meetings the matter of future expectations is raised. The anticipation of future "togetherness" with our partners is very important.

Many are still experiencing the "hard-work" years of parenting, and look forward with the hope that there will be increasing opportunities to enjoy marital companionship, soon. Others already have empty nests, are enjoying a renewed sense of freedom and the anticipation of retirement.

For all of us, this anticipation no longer seems as joyous as it once was. Hearts feel a bit heavy. Worry slightly furrows the brows of those who are slipping through the years towards retirement. Many feel that the years, rather than maintaining mutuality and shared interest, have uncovered difference and division, and, outside of shared ownership and responsibility, shared interests have evaporated away, or are buried so deep they seem unreachable.

It's hard to find the words to adequately describe this feeling, and the fear or grief that threatens to well up and overwhelm. There is no word to soothe this. The worry is real.

The only hope I can possibly raise is to remember that somewhere along the way, someone told us to try and go back and find what brought us together with our partners in the first place. That common interest or shared experience that our friendship developed around originally, when love began to spark. There is no easy suggestion as to how to do that. Re-discovering that shared interest could seem an elusive task to achieve, but may be the only way of simplifying life, and helping us discover what's really important to us. The practicalities and realities of surviving every day may seem to constantly strangle out any hope of rediscovering or enjoying those shared interests, but our thoughts can begin to explore the possibilities, and give us some hope, for today.

Recently, I've been made aware of some Couple Counselling material by a guy named John Gottman. I know very little about it, but I have begun to explore some of his concepts, which are quite interesting, particularly around predicting divorce. He says that the foundation of his approach to help a marriage survive and/or revive is to "strengthen the friendship that is at the heart of any marriage".

A thoughtful hope for weary hearts? ... Carol Grigg, November 2009

How we think

Over the years since our support group has been operating we have been privileged to have the support of several wonderful psychologists. One of these psychologists is Eleanor Gittins who has educated us on many topics and helped us to gain more understanding of Asperger's Syndrome and how it affects relationships.

In one of Eleanor's presentations she explained to us the difference in cognitive processing between "neurotypical" and "Asperger Syndrome", drawing on information from Donna Williams' Book "Exposure Anxiety" (2003).

Cognitive Processing in Asperger Syndrome involves:

- Interpretive processing at the level of the literal, with some intermittent processing beyond.
- General single tracking processing with some information processing delay.
- Lack of simultaneous sense of self and other, particularly in social interaction initiated by another.
- Cognitive Processing in Neurotypicals involves:
- Interpretive processing beyond literal to personal, relevant, specific and abstract relating.
- Multi-tracking without significant processing delay.
- Ability to maintain, seek and enjoy emotional/social interaction with another.
- Generally able to maintain a simultaneous sense of self and other in social relating.

(Hope you'll find this interesting and helpful. Carol, June 2010)

Knowing what we do

We, as partners, provide an invaluable service for our Asperger partners.

Now ... we need to remember that they typically will not acknowledge this, and may even be incensed at the suggestion because they will not be able to recognize the many ways we are doing this.

The desire to be acknowledged for what we do is absolutely normal and human. However, we must resist the urge to rub it in our partners' faces, bring it to their attention, badger or shame them over it. But quietly we know. Others in our groups and on our mailing lists know. We know that what we are doing is helping to keep our partners in orbit, functioning in life as constructively as possible, and of course we're trying to keep our families safely on track as well, which provides enormous motivation.

I am drawing attention to this concept of "rendering a service" in this way because I believe it is a positive way of looking at what we find ourselves doing to help make another person's life liveable and productive.

However, as always, I encourage you to remember your own boundaries and limitations. . .

Boundaries and limitations which, if we go beyond will deplete us of emotional, mental and physical energy that will leave us short for sustaining our own life and well-being, now and for the future, and also our children's lives, now and for the future.

There is a principle in the Bible about helping to share the burdens of another during a time of need, without taking over and carrying their entire load for them in an ongoing way. Carrying another's load for them encourages irresponsibility on their part, at the expense of another (us).   It allows them to use the resources of another to further their own interests and nurture themselves in a way they should be doing for themselves as adults.

As always, professional guidance is recommended, particularly in this case in relation to boundaries.

Carol (May 2010)

Negotiating for change

At our August support group meeting we had a discussion on practical relationship strategies that have worked. I noted a couple of interesting situations raised in the discussion, particularly significant because they were consistent with other feedback I've been receiving from partners by email and phone.

The first one was that quite a few partners are now reporting progress in their relationships at home after waiting patiently for considerable lengths of time, sometimes several years. It seems the secret is in the following:

- Sowing the seed of suggestion with their AS (suspected) partner
- Calmly and firmly pursuing information and support for their own sake
- Adjusting personal expectations & attitudes
- Suggesting professional consultation
- Not being in their face
- Just quietly waiting.

I hope this may give hope to those who still despair.

The other thing that could give hope to partners is that a number of women shared about situations where they've carefully and calmly planned towards either issuing an ultimatum to their partners or insisting on pursuing a pathway or goal that was important to their own personal development or well-being. They were prepared for a reaction, and weathered this through, but remained calmly determined that change needed to take place, for both partners' sakes, and also the family.

One example was a marital separation, which was carefully planned, and clear instructions given about what was expected from the AS partner. Failure resulted in actual separation, and now the AS partner is co-operating with her conditions in order to restore the relationship.

Another partner insists on taking a holiday on her own each year, which she plans carefully and enjoys looking forward to.

Another partner decided she was going to pursue further education in a chosen field, and followed this through.

Another partner presented in a logical manner to her AS husband that it was clear she was the cause of his anger, that the anger needed to stop, so therefore she would need to leave in order for this to happen. He responded positively & change has begun for them.

There were other examples shared as well, and I do plan to distribute a more comprehensive list in the near future.

What stood out to us was that the AS partners of these women, whilst reacting badly & intimidatingly at first, did in time settle down and accept the decisions of their partners, responding in most cases to clear-cut instructions or statements that were given calmly and firmly and were not negotiable.

It was stressed in the meeting that it is never ok to regularly threaten to leave a relationship; in fact, this is emotional blackmail.

The decision to leave should never be taken or talked about lightly. If you do decide to threaten a separation, it is imperative to describe what you expect from your partner, set a time frame, and then follow through and leave if they do not meet your conditions.

Always remember however to be realistic in what you expect, seeking professional guidance in order to manage the crisis carefully and wisely.

Carol (September 2011)

Oh to be heard and believed

"Being heard by another person greatly influences the way all of us think about ourselves and organise our lives."

I read this comment in some Course material I was studying and couldn't help but think how true this is for us.

Lately (mid 2009), there has been much trouble and unrest in the online parts of the Asperger & Neurotypical communities. Groups like ours have been accused of stereotyping as abusive all people with Asperger's Syndrome, we've been accused of being "hate groups" and "Cassandra Cults" and many incorrect assumptions have been made about what ASPIA is doing.

It is true that our group represents only troubled relationships, and that therefore we are only observing negative examples of AS/NT relationships. What is also true though is that the partners who attend our meetings have been struggling for years with a dynamic in their relationship that they did not understand and did not know how to respond to. The discovery of Asperger's Syndrome seems to have brought the clue that was missing, or removed the cork from the bottle, and many are now finding that they are beginning to be able to emerge from the tangle of confusion that has characterised their marital relationship and family life up to this present time.

We are not blaming all the relationship problems on the partner who has Asperger's Syndrome. In virtually every case the person with Asperger's Syndrome has not been aware of Asperger's Syndrome either and they have struggled with their own confusion. No-one is saying that the non-Asperger partner is innocent of contributing to the relationship difficulties. Experience has shown us that once the non-Asperger partner is believed and validated they are then emotionally able to explore their own issues as well.

We believe that awareness begins to make the difference. Then with the right information and support, combined with mutual participation to find solutions, many NT/AS couples can begin their own journey towards a more mutually satisfying level of fulfilment within the relationship.

This requires honesty and a desire for growth and change by both partners, not just the non-Asperger partner. Carol Grigg, June 2009

Out of the mouths of …

From time to time I am stopped in my tracks by the "down to earth" insights my own children express in relation to their own experience in a family affected by Asperger's Syndrome.

Recently my 12 year old son compared his childhood experience with an Asperger father to that of the concept of the "Hole in the Wall" Game Show on Pay TV.

In this game, if the contestants are able to contort their bodies to match the shaped hole in the wall, and manoeuvre their bodies in this shape safely through the hole as the wall passes over them, they avoid ending up in the plunge pool.

My son summarised his comparison with the words "Mum eventually got a cramp … and I couldn't hold my handstand for long enough".

Carol Grigg, February 2009

Perceptions of conflict

Our September meeting continued the theme of useful hints and stress-saving strategies for everyday situations in a relationship with a partner with Asperger's Syndrome.

Several more suggestions were made, but in concluding, one of our group members reminded us of a very useful and simple comment made by one of our most supportive Psychologists Jeroen Decates, which is that in relationships and life "typical people want to be happy, whereas people with Asperger's Syndrome want an absence of conflict". Therefore, absence of conflict may be the equivalent of "happiness" for them.

We went on to discuss that for someone with AS, things like a request from us, sickness in the family, a less than perfect performance or outcome, or something they can't fix, control or manage could actually mean "conflict" for them. They actually may not have the verbal, cognitive or emotional tools to be able to respond adequately or appropriately to these situations of "conflict", hence the reactions we find so confusing and distressing, and the sense that there are so many barriers getting in the way of managing or resolving issues in the relationship and home.

Jeroen also reminds us frequently that Asperger's Syndrome and anxiety go hand in hand. Increased anxiety can lead to a strengthening of Asperger traits and behaviours.

Carol Grigg (October 2011)

Pressing the pause button

When faced with a conflict situation, try to pause, think, and pull back.

It is virtually a foregone conclusion that if we pursue our case at that point, the situation will almost certainly escalate and deteriorate into something that we cannot resolve and that will cause more stress and desperation for ourselves, as well as the other person.

When in conflict with someone with Asperger's Syndrome we need to fight back our natural inclination to produce more reasons and arguments and expand our case. We need to simplify rather than complicate. Narrow down rather than expand. Stick to the one point. Deal with one issue at a time. Stay calm, use logic, eliminate emotion or emotional responses. Pause and come back to it later if emotions begin to escalate.

Try to pre-organise some signals and time frames with your partner for "time out". Yes, the frustration is high, and it feels once again like we are the one having to take responsibility for the hard work, but what's the point of beating your head against a brick wall? This only brings more pain and distress to yourself, and doesn't bring any solutions to the situation.

By escalating emotionally, expanding our argument and intensifying the situation, we are going to force the AS person into a "can't cope" and "can't comprehend" state. We will overwhelm them. Some of them will shut down at this point and disengage – which infuriates us further. Others will meltdown and become enraged, which isn't safe for anyone. They may just do whatever works to make us back off and shut up. No resolution, and no hope of resolution.

In time, once we've demonstrated a new and measured approach to conflict, our partners may stay engaged for longer and some discussion may be able to take place. While ever there's a threat of emotional escalation, the AS person is more than likely to run for cover, and we will be left with rage and frustration. Physically and emotionally this is terribly destructive for us and it is vitally important for our health and well-being to minimise these situations as much as possible.

Choose your battles, and manage them safely, for your own sake as much as anyone's. Maybe get help, talk to a professional about specific strategies.

And don't forget that communicating via email can eliminate much of the "emotional atmosphere" that takes place around face to face discussion and arguments. People with AS have trouble processing words, meaning, facial expression, eye contact, body language, tone of voice, emotion – all at once. Cut down the channels. It's worth a try.

...Carol (April 2010)

Reflecting with hindsight

Recently, an Aspie who is dear to me was given some feedback about himself from a friend who he'd known for 15 years and who he trusted and respected very much. The feedback was that she'd always found him to be an "intense" person. It wasn't said in a critical way, but in a matter of fact way that was consistent with the context of the conversation. It was interesting to watch his response at the time, and a privilege to be the one he confided in later when he'd had time to ponder and process the comment.

Before I share his response, I think it's important for us to pause and note that there was a time delay before he was able to respond, but encouraging that he was able to go through a process of thinking about what was said, self-reflecting, coming to his own understanding and then verbalizing what he believed was the reason or explanation for the characteristic his friend had commented about.

He began his explanation by saying "You know how when Aspies enter a new situation they don't typically pick up on the clues and cues around them to know how to behave and what to say?" I acknowledged this. He said that this is how it is for him, so he has to look for information deliberately, and that the intensity his friend had noticed about him was probably how he came across while he went through the process of scanning desperately for information so that he would know how to behave and what to say in that context.

I thought this was a very fair and reasonable comment, and I found it really helped me to further understand some of those AS characteristics and moments I've found so confusing over the years.

When you think about it, if you add the fact that AS people generally don't generalize (ie, transfer learned behaviour from one situation to another situation that is similar but not the same), then they are going through this deliberate scanning process constantly, looking for information that will guide them in how to behave and what to say.

Exhausting I would say. Anxiety laden in fact, when you think about how afraid they are of making a mistake or getting it "wrong".

Writing this has also directed my thoughts to those moments we all talk about when our partners respond quickly with a defense or rationalisation about their behaviour that just doesn't sit true with us. Perhaps their response has more to do with an inability to think and reflect on the spot, clutching at straws, trying to save face and an attempt to deflect a comment, feedback or criticism they don't understand and need time to think about and process.

Perhaps we could help them and help ourselves by not taking to heart or judging instantly the words they speak in haste, and by recognizing that they do need that extra time to process and reflect.

Like I said in my first paragraph, I felt very privileged to hear the response later, because so often we don't hear back from them and are never quite sure what they are thinking.

Perhaps they take on board more than we think. Carol (November 2011)

Relationship essentials

There are two things that are essential for an Asperger marriage to survive, recover or grow.

First is that the person with Asperger's Syndrome be willing to explore and accept the existence of Asperger's Syndrome in their personality and their relationship, and hopefully seek professional guidance.

People with AS tend to cope better and help their partners and families cope better when they are pro-active in understanding and managing their AS characteristics better. I know that many partners reading this carry a lot of grief over the hope of this happening for their relationship.

Second, the non-Asperger partner must stop believing that their partner will become neurotypical if they just learn about AS, "get it", accept it, get diagnosed or if we try hard enough to convince them.

It is imperative for non-AS partners to continue to learn and thoroughly understand the facts about AS and how it is manifesting in their own relationship. Then we have to allow our minds to make a shift into accepting the AS, that it is here to stay and that change will be slow and limited, even with the most co-operative AS partner.

Some great words of advice from a parent training course (123 Magic & Emotion Coaching) are to "avoid too much talk, and too much emotion" when dealing with our children.

This is important advice for adult relationships too, but particularly when Asperger's Syndrome is present, because one of the core difficulties in AS is in the processing of communication and emotions.

A good motto is: Avoid too much talk and too much emotion.

Carol Grigg (December 2011)

Remembering who we are

When partners first make contact with ASPIA, either by attending a support group meeting or phoning me, they are usually in quite a state of distress.

Energy is gone, frustration is through the roof, hope is in tatters, tears flow unchecked.

Amongst many sentiments, almost every partner expresses great sadness at the realisation they are no longer the person they used to be. The change that causes the most concern is anger. Most partners did not start out as angry people.

Most partners are, or were, quite calm, patient and caring individuals. It is very distressing to wake up one day and recognise the change, feeling powerless to dissipate or contain one's anger while personal circumstances remain unchanged and, for many, intolerable due to unresolved conflict, constant miscommunication and much anxiety.

Anger drives us to behave in ways we are later ashamed of, and guilt makes us feel even worse. Being in this state is agonising.

By the time we have reached the point of no longer feeling like the person we once were, we need help for ourselves. It will be virtually impossible to remain objective within a couple counselling context, unless and until we have had an opportunity to de-brief our own stuff, and find some clarity in the fog.

This is why ASPIA pushes the idea of self-care so strongly. If we've lost who we are, we need to find ourselves again. Attending a support group or meeting with others is very important and life changing, but we mustn't underestimate or play down the importance and value of having personal counselling for ourselves, particularly around issues of loss and grief.

Partners need to focus first on finding a pathway back to who they were. Only from that place will we be able to be true to ourselves once again and find the calmness, strength and courage to make decisions and constructive contributions to ours and our family's futures.

… Carol (December 2009)

Some thoughts shared

by Clinical Psychologist Jeroen Decates (August 2010):

Our partners may have feelings/emotions but may not be able to give meaning to what they are experiencing, attach meaning to behaviour, or be able to put the right words around this.

Our partners can't intuitively adjust to new situations or be creative about new ways of doing things.

We (non AS people) trade with social cues all the time.

AS people may learn mechanically, not because they know or feel something.

For AS people a state of contentment is the absence of conflict.

For non-AS people a state of contentment is happiness.

"Happiness" may not mean to an AS person what it means to us.

An AS person may perceive that the pursuit or achievement of "happiness" as we define it, could in fact introduce for them the potential for conflict with partners and family members.

AS people may be ruthlessly logical.

Recommended reading for our AS partners - Jeroen suggests Simon Baron-Cohen's book "The Essential Difference" because it doesn't have "Asperger's Syndrome" in the title, and it presents brain differences in a more "male acceptable" way.

by Clinical Psychologist Julie Peterson (September 2010):

Julie focused our attention on the importance of stretching, exercise, relaxation, meditation, affirmations.

It is crucial for partners to attend to ways of reducing their own personal anxiety and stress in order to avoid and prevent stress-related illness and disease and other breakdowns of our mortal frames and minds.

The group was encouraged to join in with Julie with some stretching, relaxation and listening exercises and many commented on feeling an immediate benefit.

by Psychologist Eleanor Gittins (2010):

A compulsion to hoard is often related to anxiety in the following ways:

- Fear of loss;
- Control the uncontrollable;
- Predictability and future order;
- Concern with error;
- Indecision
- Disorganization
- Perfectionism
- Procrastination

Other (source unknown):

"In people with Asperger Syndrome, familiar sustained attention events become increasingly favoured; while new, frequently changing (people and social) events provoke stress and tend to be avoided (or sabotaged) for their unpredictability and/or mental labour."

More helpful information (July 2011):

See Sue Larkey's helpful article about why AS people are so afraid of making mistakes, and also why they don't seem to learn from their mistakes. She calls it a difficulty with "cognitive flexibility". Copy & paste this link into your web browser:
http://clicks.aweber.com/y/ct/?l=8LpOa&m=lj2ZfjUZM2v439&b=_JP9UQ7ujIBsAlz8swFtpw

An old friend Lorna who is a mental health worker and grief counsellor made the following response to our newsletter "thoughts" last month – "…your comments … are far from bleak! They are realistic and in line with grief work and also recovery-oriented practice. Accepting the reality and feeling the pain of the loss (of the dream) are so important for moving on and healing in so many areas of life."

Jeroen Decates frequently reminds us at meetings that "Neurotypicals want to be happy; people with Asperger's Syndrome want an absence of conflict."

In our June meeting, Julie Peterson and Steve Den Kaat used the analogy of a bucket to describe our ability to cope with everyday life and situations, explaining how the bucket of the person with Asperger's Syndrome is already almost full all of the time, and any additional stress or challenge will often cause it to overflow, with meltdowns, etc following.

They went on to explain that sometimes it is actually necessary and better if the meltdown can occur because this allows for a defusion of the frustration, and enables the person with AS to calm themselves and settle back down to a manageable level of stress again. Not pleasant for the partner or family member, as we are all very painfully aware, but Julie and Steve reminded us how important it is that we try to work on not taking these reactions and meltdowns personally, because at a high level of stress and meltdown, everyone becomes irrational and IQ levels drop, including the person with AS.

Julie & Steve did some wonderful role plays to demonstrate the build-up to a meltdown between an NT and AS couple, and then alternatives to try and avoid a situation reaching meltdown.

Info about the link between emotions and behaviour (not AS specific, but interesting)

"Each of the four basic emotions has cognitive (perceptual) and behavioural correlates.

Sadness is evoked when there is a perception of defeat, loss or deprivation. The behavioural consequence is to withdraw.

Elation follows from perceived gain and reinforces activity toward the goal.

Anxiety is triggered by perceived vulnerability and threat, and the behavioural consequence is to withdraw, "freeze", or prepare for defense.

Anger, in contrast, is directed to the offensive qualities of the threat, and the behavioural inclination is to attack."

(Counselling Diploma study notes - Cognitive Behaviour Therapy, AIPC.)

A few words about what goes on in our support group meetings

It could be understandable that the Asperger partners of those who attend our meetings, may fear that we are "Aspie bashers" and that we are trying to break up Asperger marriages.

Rather than harming our marriages, those who attend our meetings know that most of the partners who attend our meetings are looking for ways to stay with their marriages, and in the majority of cases they do. Our aim is to support partners within their relationships, not support them to leave their relationships, unless this is what an individual partner believes that he/she needs to do, for their own reasons.

We have sought to bring frequent professional input and education into our meetings so that partners can learn more about AS, understand their AS partners and find ways to ease the miscommunication and conflict that is a dominant characteristic in their relationship.

We are also building up an excellent library of books that all focus on understanding Asperger's Syndrome & practical suggestions for a more successful relationship.

For many partners, just gaining some understanding makes all the difference because they can then make adjustments to their expectations of themselves, their partner and their relationship, and live more at peace within that. We see the difference on their faces from one month to the next as they begin to come to terms with their own reality and find ways to respect themselves better.

For some the help has come too late. The long-term confusion, lack of awareness of AS, absence of support and intervention and layers of unresolved issues have all taken too great a toll. The partner has to face the reality that to hold the relationship together any longer could mean the loss of their own emotional and physical health and well-being permanently. In many cases it is the needs of the children that must become the priority, and be balanced against the ongoing effort required to save the struggling marriage.

Some who previously separated have chosen to return to the relationship on new or refreshingly unconventional terms, including partial separation. This may enable them to enjoy "togetherness" in activities that they enjoy, but also to enjoy activities as individuals as well.

Some continue on in the difficult circumstances and are just glad to have our newsletters or a place like our ASPIA meetings to receive validation and be reminded of their own value.

The best situations are where the partner with Asperger's Syndrome is willing to accept their AS and co-operate with professional advice and the guidance of their partner.

Every non-AS partner would wish for this, and it is the key that would make a beautiful difference in every situation.

Yes, ASPIA meetings are a place for sharing our difficulties, but this enables partners to de-brief and receive validation – all in the context of confidentiality and relative anonymity.

Once we have had an opportunity to "get things off our chest", many are then ready and able to take on board the positives of new learning that will help us approach our relationships with renewed energy and hope.

My thoughts are with you all, Carol (July 2008)

A sense of belonging

"All of us who attend meetings are feeling the benefit of having our own connecting point where we can talk frankly about our struggles and breakthroughs.

It's like finding our own "tribe", like we belong."

Carol, Dec 2008/Jan 2009

When Difference Divides

While ploughing through some reading material for my Diploma of Professional Counselling (AIPC) I constantly come across the most interesting thoughts and theories, many of which I'd love to share in our newsletters.

The latest gem I came across is a definition of Stages 6 & 7 of ego development by psychodynamic theorist Jane Loevinger. These stages are deemed to be the stages of adulthood. I'm sure you'll find these as interesting as I did:

Stage 6 Autonomy – The ego is autonomous when it can tolerate, rather than condemn, opposing opinions and viewpoints. During this stage, respect is accorded to others who hold differing convictions and principles.

Stage 7 Integration – This stage represents a full acceptance of who one is in terms of ego development. This includes one's strengths as well as weaknesses, and one's successes as well as failures. Conflicting internal demands and the demands of others are now reconciled and tolerated. Integration in this sense implies peace with oneself, recognition of one's total being, and an appreciation of the individuality of others.

My interpretation, as I think these relate to us? My personal suspicion is that many partners were already aware of and developing these stages in our lives when we first embarked on our marital relationships.

We were clearly open to seeking out and accepting partners who were "differently interesting", holding the belief that difference would enhance the relationship rather than posing a threat to future function and happiness; we were secure in who we were, then.

Our belief also included the assumption that the marital context would be one of mutual appreciation and tolerance, reciprocity of respect and adaptability, and embracing of the differences between us to create a deeply interesting, mature and satisfying union.

Many of us still hang on to our belief in this potential, but feel locked into a state of isolation and disconnect inside of our relationships by the ways communication continually tangles up into a conflicting gridlock of meanings and interpretations that create alienation and frustration.

Sadly and helplessly, difference has progressively led to division rather than mutual respect and embrace.

As a conclusion, perhaps we can just use these definitions of adulthood as a benchmark for ourselves, to help us reclaim and maintain our own physchological well-being as truly autonomous and integrated individuals, in spite of our circumstances. Be who you are, or were, and go on from there.

As always, I strongly recommend securing professional counselling in order to regain and retain perspective, and don't forget our group's self-care suggestions listed on the website: http://www.aspia.org.au/pdf/2009/ASPIASelf-CareSuggestions6June09.pdf   (copy & paste this link into your web browser)

Carol (May 2011)

Words and tone

In last month's Newsletter I discussed a particular aspect of communication, and this month I find myself pondering yet another aspect of communication. After all, some say that Asperger's Syndrome is primarily a disorder of communication, so it makes sense to look at all the ways our communication is affected.

What I've noticed specifically in some interactions this past month is how sensitive an Asperger person can be to the way we communicate with them. They notice and seem to over-react to the tone in our voice, the attitude they perceive we are expressing, the words we use and the intensity of our approach. It seems they almost always seem to perceive that we are attacking them, even when we feel we are just seeking to discuss a matter objectively, or make factual comments about a situation to which they are contributing; matters and situations that affect us or the family in significant ways, and that we need to create some dialogue around for the purpose of finding solutions or a pathway forward.

For so many, problems with communication create an impasse in the relationship or family situation and we have no idea how to work around all the technicalities that seem to jam up the cogs. All of us are loathe to criticize or attack our partners unjustly, but we know that the impasses are still happening even when we've gone to great lengths to form our words and attitudes carefully and non-judgmentally. It is easy to want to give up or stop trying so hard out of exasperation and a sense of hopelessness.

Added to this then is what we perceive is a great injustice when our Asperger loved ones seem to be insensitive towards us with their own tone, words, attitudes and intensity. It's easy to feel like there are two sets of rules and we can become very resentful over this. We feel like our own mouths have been stopped, but that we are unable to place effective boundaries in place around the ways they communicate with us that are emotionally harmful.

Before I get your hopes up too high, I have to say I haven't worked out what to do about this yet as it seems to come with the territory, but it's probably still very important for us not to just give up in exasperation or start "treating them the way they treat us" to try to teach them what it feels like, because that's a pathway that leads to nowhere, and it doesn't make us feel any better. In fact, it more than likely will just make things worse because our AS loved one will not understand why our attitudes have deteriorated so much or why we seem like we're out to get them.

You see, what I have realized is that they just do not seem to perceive how they're coming across. This instinct and the ability to moderate their responses just don't seem to be taking place, as much as it's so hard for us to get our heads around. I have no doubt that some of them learn to use an aggressive manner of communication because they've observed its effectiveness in securing the outcome they desire, but I actually believe in many instances that the reactions are based more on how important or urgent the matter is to them, or how fearful or stressed they are, rather than out of intent to cut us down or hurt us personally.

I have heard that many with Aspergers are quite distressed in hindsight when they realise how much they've hurt someone's feelings, but they may not be able to convey this to us or know how to avoid it another time. Awareness of how their words and actions are impacting on us requires instantaneous empathy and imagination which perhaps are additional dimensions that their minds cannot hold at the same time.

Remember they cannot hold awareness in their minds about what's happening for them and what's happening for us, simultaneously. That is part of Asperger's Syndrome.

When things are calm, perhaps it could be useful to try and provide some illustrations to the AS person that relate to the saying: "You don't need a ten tonne crane to lift a feather." Maybe describe the contrast between a tack hammer and a sledge hammer or a candle and a blowtorch. These concepts may be best presented in writing, using some describing words around how the sledge hammer or blowtorch make you feel, but try to remain logical and objective and keep the emotional terminology simple.

Carol (March 2011)

Section 5 Words fail us - Advocacy and Representation

"Without an Understanding of Asperger's Syndrome, people make a moral judgment." Tony Attwood, 13 August 2009

Words Fail Us

A significant and traumatic part of every partner's story includes the years of being disbelieved, misjudged or abandoned when professional help or church, peer or family support was sought.

The experience of being disbelieved and misjudged, often repeatedly, multiplied many times over the distress and confusion we were living in our personal lives and led many of us on the dangerous and downward spiralling journey of self-doubt towards depression and a host of other dark places.

The importance of validation has been mentioned and reinforced many times over in this book because of its importance in helping us to claw back a sense of confidence again in our own credibility.

Some of us testify to "Divine Guidance" in our search for the truth, and will remain grateful for this guidance to our dying day, and even beyond I'm sure.

Whilst most of us have been privileged to find professionals now who "get it", there is still distress and anxiety at the realization that right across society there are still a great many organisations, government or non-government, educational or religious, legal or welfare, etc who still do not understand enough about Asperger's Syndrome in adults to recognize or identify the characteristics or behaviours when they are impacting significantly on a situation at hand.

This raises a significant risk of discrimination or injustice being carried out towards not only the individuals with Asperger's Syndrome themselves, but also to their partners, children, siblings or parents.

I have noted a number of times, with a little cynicism I must confess, that our movie and TV producers these days seem to "get" Asperger's Syndrome more accurately than a great number of health professionals around the world who, rather than being the empathic first base of identification and referral or diagnosis, they let another seeking soul slip unheard and invalidated through to the keeper for another day and another professional to pick up the pieces another year or so down the track of personal crisis.

Trying to put a description of Asperger's Syndrome into a nutshell is still an impossibility due to its complexity and layers and the variation in meanings that are placed around characteristic behaviours. Written information still tends to be comprehensive and wordy. The pages that follow here are provided with the hope that they may assist you to find the words to describe or explain to others what Asperger's Syndrome means for you and your family. Carol, March 2012

Misjudged

"Without an understanding of Asperger's Syndrome people make a moral judgment" (Tony Attwood, 13 August 2009)

I was present when Tony Attwood made this comment during one of his recent presentations, and it has continued to resound through my whole being ever since. He was referring particularly to what happens to people with Asperger's Syndrome when society doesn't understand them or their behaviours.

On thinking it through though, I believe this can also apply to the experience of a partner, parent or other family member.

People not only judge the person with Asperger's Syndrome, they judge family members too as somehow having contributed to, caused or neglected to prevent the behaviour in some way, and the family member is made to share the shunning, judgment and isolation that the AS person experiences.

Ironically, when we've tried to get help or tell our story we're disbelieved or discredited, and judged as being malicious or neurotic.

Increased awareness of Asperger's Syndrome within society is so vitally important. It makes all the difference when behaviours and situations are viewed through the "lens" of understanding of Asperger's Syndrome. Carol Grigg (September 2009)

Describing the Characteristics of Asperger's Syndrome within Marital and Family Situations (May be useful when care professionals or welfare workers need to be involved)

Clinical descriptions of Asperger's Syndrome are not written in every-day language and are difficult to translate into how people with Asperger's Syndrome are actually experienced by others in day-to-day real-life situations, particularly by their partners in a marriage or long-term relationship, or by children, parents or siblings in a family situation.

Indeed, clinical descriptions also don't adequately convey what the person with Asperger's Syndrome is experiencing at a human level.

Those who are diagnosed with Asperger's Syndrome tend to have difficulty discerning how their words and actions are experienced by others, and so are often unable to describe or even acknowledge the ways they are coming across.

Family members, including partners and children, have often sought help from the care professions, other family members and sometimes even the authorities, but find themselves typically disbelieved and even judged as making malicious accusations.

This document was written in response to an awareness of a number of situations of this nature, where families may have either sought help from care or welfare agencies, or inadvertently come to the attention of these agencies, but have found that interventions have proved either traumatic, futile or even destructive to all family members involved. Family members often find that their testimonies are disbelieved or discredited, and resulting interventions may in fact be discriminatory in the light of the fact that Asperger's Syndrome is a developmental disability, and often hereditary.

It is extremely important for care and welfare professions to recognise the often hidden or misleading aspects of Asperger's Syndrome and therefore adjust their first line of approach when working with families in general.

Descriptions of some of the more significant characteristics that impact on family life are as follows:

1. People with Asperger's Syndrome tend to have a need for control.

This may be over:

- their partner
- children or other family members
- home routines
- social life
- family values
- activities
- finances
- belongings
- religion
- education choices,
- etc.

Reasons for this can be as follows:

- High anxiety
- a need for predictability and order
- difficulty with change of any kind
- difficulty sustaining healthy attachments
- belief that own values are the only ones to hold
- fear of exposure
- absolute need for their routines or prescribed methods to be used in all aspects of household functioning and activities
- inability to accommodate the thoughts and values of other people
- a need to "save face"
- etc.

Behaviours they may display or learn to use to ensure control (intimidating to others):

- Verbal abuse
- Blame
- criticism
- bullying
- oppositional behaviour
- vindictiveness, manipulation
- emotional blackmail
- withdrawal or "shut-downs"
- rage/emotional escalation or "melt-downs"
- avoidance/running away
- panic attacks
- withholding of finances
- prevention of opportunities
- helplessness and playing "victim"
- accusations of disloyalty or being against them
- disrespect for authority,
- threats
- harassment
- stalking
- suicide threats
- violence
- intrusiveness
- avoidance or refusal of responsibility.

Note: It is important to mention that people with AS seem to fall into two fairly distinct categories of expression, with very little "in between". Some can be extremely passive, using withdrawal and "passive aggressive" types of behaviours such as resistance, refusal, avoidance, etc. Others can be aggressive and outward in their methods of maintaining control. These behaviours will typically be hidden in public.

2. People with Asperger's Syndrome are usually very intelligent and can be quite articulate.

This can be very misleading as it gives the impression of someone who's credible, stable and able to follow through on undertakings.

It is not only the family members who are disadvantaged as a result of this misleading aspect, but also the person who has Asperger's Syndrome because they and the family can then be refused the supports or compassionate interventions they so desperately need and deserve.

3. People with Asperger's Syndrome have communication difficulties.

These are subtle at first, and not suspected, due to verbal ability and intelligence.

- Asperger's Syndrome prevents people accurately interpreting verbal communication.
- Mental processing of a message is slow, so there may be gaps in what they hear.
- They have a tendency to interpret messages literally and may miss implied meanings.
- They may have trouble forming an acceptable answer within a reasonable time frame.
- Their anxiety increases and their ability to interpret decreases as we add emotion, tone change, expression, body language, facial expression and force to our message.
- They often interpret our attempts to discuss situations as a personal attack on them, resulting in suspicion, resistance, hostility, opposition, retaliation and shutdowns/meltdowns.
- These difficulties with communication can lead to the development of hostility and suspicion for all parties involved due to misunderstandings of what's taking place. These communication difficulties also thwart or limit the effectiveness of traditional counselling or mediation efforts.
- People with Asperger's Syndrome need to be given logical and practical strategies and steps to follow rather than advice, and those who work with them need to have a calm and clear-cut method of approach.

4. People with Asperger's Syndrome seem to be perceiving and experiencing situations differently to typical people.

This may include the following:

- A heightened sensitivity to light, noise, smell, touch and taste which can overwhelm and distract them, causing elevated anxiety, avoidance of situations and inability to cope;
- Different logic and focus leading to different priorities which can cause families to feel that the family member with Asperger's Syndrome is more concerned about the physical environment, routines, special interests, possessions or values than with the needs and well-being of the human beings around them.

5. People with Asperger's Syndrome are not easily able to read other people and respond empathically in the moment, nor are they aware of the impact that their own attitudes and behaviours may be having on those around them.

These deficits can lead to behaviours that may be perceived by others as:

- Inappropriate
- Neglectful
- Rude
- Insensitive
- Risky
- causing deprivation
- cruel
- embarrassing
- callous
- intrusive

- overwhelming
- arrogant
- self-centred
- etc.

An understanding of Asperger's Syndrome can enable onlookers to avoid making moral judgments about the individual's character in these situations.

Other important points to note:

- People with Asperger's Syndrome are at high risk for Anxiety and Depression.
- It is not uncommon for people with Asperger's Syndrome to consider or attempt suicide.
- Asperger's Syndrome is being diagnosed in people who may also have another condition such as Bipolar Disorder, ADD, ADHD, Borderline Personality Disorder, Oppositional Defiant Disorder, Tourette's Syndrome, Anxiety, Depression, etc.

This document has been prepared as a guide only. Readers are encouraged to seek professional guidance from Care professionals who can demonstrate an extensive clinical experience working with adults with Asperger's Syndrome and their families. See ASPIA's website for a list of recommended Clinicians.

Just present what is …

A few months ago I mentioned I had secured an opportunity to speak with a representative of our Department of Community Services on the issues surrounding families affected by Asperger's Syndrome.

I asked people on our mailing list to provide me with some real-life examples or experiences that I could include in my presentation. I am very glad to report that I actually had two opportunities to speak with two different women in management positions within the department. They were both very open and receptive to the things I shared, and responded with some very down-to-earth practical ideas. In fact, they both seemed to "get it", showing significant understanding of Asperger's Syndrome. It is to be hoped in time that this knowledge will filter down to the Case Workers who manage families at the front-line in the community.

One of the key threads that emerged from these talks is that, whether our situation involves Asperger's Syndrome or not, if our children are being significantly impacted on by parenting difficulties or our marital issues and/or conflict, then we have a responsibility to our children to seek help from an organisation that offers parenting support, such as Relationships Australia or Centacare, etc.

By doing this we are creating a professional record. If the matters are serious, we may also need to create a record of having sought legal advice.

If you have serious issues, do not keep avoiding, thinking the troubles will go away, or that you can't prove Asperger's Syndrome. You may leave yourself and your children vulnerable to unjust intervention or defeat in Court further down the track unless you take some responsibility to consult with appropriate professionals now and create a record of what is happening.

Don't try to prove that your partner or the child's other parent has Asperger's Syndrome. We are aware of cases now where this sadly has gone against the parent making these claims, simply because Asperger's Syndrome can be so hidden, the manifestations are easily played down or misinterpreted and our claims can appear to be made with ill-intent.

Just present "what is", describing clearly what is happening and the impact you believe it is having on your children. Demonstrate your co-operation with the guidance you are given.

Carol Grigg, March 2009

Suggested Approaches and Strategies for use with Families where Asperger's Syndrome is or may be present in an Adult and when Welfare Intervention may be needed

IMPORTANT: Avoid confrontational approach or traumatic intervention if at all possible.

- Non-Asperger parent will normally be quite responsible and emotionally capable of caring for child but needs to be heard and supported.
- Interventions need to be designed to support both parents. The non-Asperger parent needs to be heard and empowered. The Asperger parent may need mentoring and accountability.
- As mentioned above, avoid traumatic intervention if possible.
- Introduce practical supports and ensure that family is followed up, sensitively and regularly. Do not leave non-Asperger partner without support.

When approaching the person with Asperger's Syndrome, it is important to:

- Keep the emotional atmosphere calm, avoid force or high-handedness
- Use curiosity rather than criticism
- Keep communication simple, clear-cut, direct and logical, avoid ambiguity or implied meanings
- Written or visual information is more easily assimilated
- Allow time for information to sink in
- Express intentions or explain actions in order they'll be carried out
- Explain goals and steps on how to achieve the goals
- Be aware of signs of anxiety building up, back off, turn body or eyes away, give space
- Limit or narrow requests/responses rather than expand or elaborate
- When approaching other family members
- Listen and believe, take the time to discover underlying issues and history
- Explore family dynamics, may be long-term psychological abuse or control
- Partner may be the "innocent but powerless parent" (words of Children's Court Magistrate)
- Seek input from wider family, friends, GPs, therapists
- Stay involved, do not abandon partner or children, set up regular visits to maintain support and accountability, offer services and/or referral

Partner may be carrying unreasonable load of responsibility for most household matters and family well-being.

Asia Pacific Autism Conference 2009 (APAC 09), Sydney, Australia

In mid-late 2008 an invitation was distributed by the organisers of the Asia-Pacific Autism Conference of 2009 (APAC 09) to interested professionals, organisations and individuals to submit Abstract Proposals for presentations supporting the themes of the conference.

One of the Streams was "Family Life, Family Functioning and Family Resilience".

Within ASPIA we felt this topic was particularly relevant to partners and family members of adults with Asperger's Syndrome, and not just parents of children with Asperger's Syndrome.

Two of the Sub-streams "Building Resilience & Capacity" and "Navigating Care Systems" were also particularly relevant in relation to ASPIA's support work.

As was mentioned in the introduction to this Section, a significant and traumatic part of every partner's story includes the years of being disbelieved, misjudged or abandoned when professional help or church, peer or family support was sought.

When partner support began more than ten years ago, finding professionals experienced with adults and relationships was like looking for a needle in a haystack. There was no pathway into the existing Care Systems, let alone a hope for re-building personal or family resilience and capacity.

We responded to the invitation by submitting an Abstract Proposal with the title "Improved Awareness within Care Systems may help prevent Family Breakdown".

Our proposal was accepted, and was to be presented in the form of a Poster. Presenting it as a Poster suited me fine as my strengths lie in writing not public speaking. It was very exciting that we were being given this opportunity, but I instantly recognized the privilege we had been honoured with and the responsibility we had to present our concerns in as constructive and professional a manner as possible.

Hence, the following information about our Poster – the actual Abstract Proposal, my Biographical information and then the Poster content.

At the time of preparing the Poster and the supporting information it was estimated that ASPIA had gathered anecdotal evidence from the testimonials of more than 1000 Australian families, and we felt confident that the information presented in the Poster was an accurate representation of these families' experiences.

Carol Grigg, March 2012

Abstract Proposal – "Improved Awareness within Care Systems may help prevent Family Breakdown"

Stream 3: Family Life, Family Functioning and Family Resilience.

Sub-streams: Building Resilience & Capacity, Navigating Care Systems;

This submission concerns the point at which families affected by an Autism Spectrum Disorder in an adult family member seek to navigate care systems to secure appropriate intervention and support.

It is the writer's contention that many families who once stood strong and proud have experienced the erosion of family resilience and capacity due to the presence of unidentified characteristics of Asperger's Syndrome within an adult member of the family.

Many of these families have experienced further erosion of family resilience and capacity when they have been unable to secure professional help and intervention when it was needed. It is a common experience of partners that professionals and community service representatives in general everywhere are alarmingly ignorant in relation to the identification of Asperger's Syndrome in adults. As Asperger's Syndrome can affect parenting skills, some families begin to lose their capacity to cope adequately with the responsibilities of parenting, particularly if a child of the family is also affected by an ASD. For some families who are not coping, professional ignorance has also proved very destructive and led to the placement of punitive interventions and orders upon them by child protection authorities and family courts.

There is nothing more unjust than a family already called on to accept the presence of an ASD within the family, than being denied supports and interventions when they sought them, and then being punished for not being able to cope.

ASDs are a family affair. Awareness by our professional community of Asperger's Syndrome within adult relationships and parenting, and the provision of appropriate supports will ensure that families are supported to be able to re-build the resilience and capacity they began with and enable them to cope with the circumstances they have been dealt.

Carol Grigg, ASPIA INC

Biographical Information of Author

Biographical Information for Carol Grigg, Author of Advocacy Poster for APAC 09 (Asia-Pacific Autism Conference 2009, Sydney, Australia)

Emerging from 20 years of marriage to a husband with Asperger's Syndrome, and parenting five children within that environment, Carol has gone on to commence and oversee ASPIA, a support group and website for partners of adults with Asperger's Syndrome based in Sydney.

The passion that drives her is based on the desperate isolation and lack of support that eventually contributed to her own family's collapse, and the awareness that this is still happening to families today.

It is Carol's firm belief that many of these families can survive and even thrive if our care systems and professionals recognise the presence of Asperger characteristics when a family presents, and respond with careful and appropriate interventions and support.

August 2009

Poster Presented - "Improved Awareness within Care Systems may help prevent Family Breakdown"

How?

- By earlier detection of Asperger's Syndrome in adult member of family;
- By earlier provision of supports for adults affected by Asperger's Syndrome and their families.

Families that once stood strong and proud, have experienced erosion of resilience and capacity due to the presence of unidentified characteristics of Asperger's Syndrome within an adult member of the family.

Why?

- No prior awareness or identification of neurological difference;
- Typical assumptions and expectations of relationships and family life;
- No knowledge of how to respond or negotiate effectively within marital or family situation when neurological difference is present;
- Professional help has often proved ineffective because our care systems are largely unaware and therefore unable to recognise the signs of Asperger's Syndrome being present in an adult member of a family.
- Barriers to receiving help
- family doesn't know about Asperger's Syndrome;
- they can't adequately describe what is taking place in the family situation;
- they fear they won't be believed;
- adult with Asperger's Syndrome may be able to mask their difficulties when away from home;
- adult with Asperger's Syndrome may be unaware of the extent or impact of their difficulties on their own life or their family;
- care systems don't know enough about Asperger's Syndrome and may interpret or assess problems incorrectly;
- appropriate supports and services are simply not available.

Autism Spectrum Disorders are a Family Affair

Without support and professional guidance, adults with Asperger's Syndrome and their partners may lose resilience and the capacity to cope adequately with the challenges of their relationship and parenting, particularly if they have a child with an Autism Spectrum Disorder as well.

"Without an understanding of Asperger's Syndrome, people make a moral judgment."
(Tony Attwood, 13 August 2009)

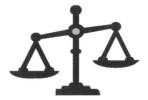

There is nothing more unjust than a family already called on to accept the presence of an Autism Spectrum Disorder within the family, being denied supports and interventions when sought, and then punished or judged for not being able to cope.

Improved awareness within our care systems in relation to Asperger's Syndrome in adult relationships and parenting, and the provision of appropriate supports or referrals, will ensure that families are assisted to re-build the resilience and capacity they began with and enable them to cope better with the circumstances they have been dealt.

(The information presented in this leaflet (above) is based on the testimonials of more than 1000 Australian families. Written and presented as a Poster for APAC 09 by Carol Grigg, Co-Founder and President of ASPIA INC (Asperger Syndrome Partner Information Australia Incorporated)

ASPIA has been conducting support group meetings and educational workshops in Sydney since 2003, as well as providing a helpline and website. Visit www.aspia.org.au or email info@aspia.org.au

Poster - Extended Version: "Improved Awareness within Care Systems may help prevent Family Breakdown"

How?

- By earlier detection of Asperger's Syndrome in adult member of family;
- By earlier provision of supports for adults affected by Asperger's Syndrome and their families.

Families that once stood strong and proud, have experienced erosion of resilience and capacity due to the presence of unidentified characteristics of Asperger's Syndrome within an adult member of the family.

Why?

- No prior awareness or identification of neurological difference;
- Typical assumptions and expectations of relationships and family life;
- No knowledge of how to respond or negotiate effectively within marital or family situation when neurological difference is present;
- Professional help has often proved ineffective because our care systems are largely unaware and therefore unable to recognise the signs of Asperger's Syndrome being present in an adult member of a family.

What?

Possible indicators of Asperger's Syndrome could include:

- Heightened sensitivity to sounds, sights, touch, food texture & tastes, scents & smells, emotional atmosphere;
- Aversion to or reduced capacity to cope with crowds or extended social interaction, noise & chaos, change & unpredictability, verbal confrontation & emotional situations;
- Anxiety;
- Depression;
- Collecting, hoarding, narrow obsessive interests;
- Tendency to rely on order, routines and rules, without flexibility;
- Unusual priorities;
- Rapid changes in mood and emotion;
- Awkwardness with people and some social situations;
- Communication differences and difficulties. (see following box)
- Difficulties and differences in communication can include:
- misunderstanding others and being misunderstood;
- misinterpretation of meaning;
- missing and misreading verbal and non-verbal signals;
- lacking language to explain or describe thoughts, feelings, experiences;
- strong ability to remember and recount factual information;
- interpreting communication and words literally;
- missing implied meanings and hints;
- focus on word usage and spelling rather than gist and meaning;
- may talk at length on topic of special interest.

Erosion of Family Resilience and Capacity

Undetected Asperger's Syndrome may cause erosion of family resilience and capacity in the following ways:

- confusion and lack of knowledge about how to respond;
- communication difficulties impede negotiation & conflict resolution;
- increased anxiety for all family members;
- adult with AS may impose own routines and preferences on others, particularly as personal anxiety increases;
- frustration and fear;
- fractured or fragile relationships between family members;
- stress and exhaustion;
- mental health problems, particularly chronic anxiety and depression;
- as personal and family demands increase, adult with AS may either attempt to exert more control within the household or lose the capacity or will to sustain responsibilities, placing greater strain on the partner;
- deterioration in parenting capacity;
- loss of employment or employment opportunities;
- social isolation;

Autism Spectrum Disorders may be a family affair

When a child is diagnosed with an Autism Spectrum Disorder, some families then go on to discover that one or both parents may also have some characteristics of Asperger's Syndrome, or vice versa. Parenting in this day and age is challenging for any parent, but particularly so if a child has a disorder or disability. Naturally, the challenge increases if one or both parents also have difficulties that could impact on their capacity to cope. Timely and appropriate intervention and support could make all the difference to a family's ability to cope, and may prevent the tragic and traumatic imposing of punitive interventions and Court Orders separating parents and children that can occur as a result of personal or family breakdown, particularly if Welfare and Court systems do not understand Asperger's Syndrome either.

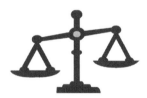

There is nothing more unjust than a family already called on to accept the presence of an Autism Spectrum Disorder within the family, being denied supports and interventions when sought, and then punished for not being able to cope.

"Without an understanding of Asperger's Syndrome, people make a moral judgment."
(Tony Attwood, 13 August 2009

Family Breakdown

<u>How</u>?

When any person or family lives with long-term confusion, conflict and stress, and is unable to access help when needed or sought, they can become frustrated and overwhelmed leading to the possibility of unfortunate and serious consequences, such as:

- inability to cope;
- anger and rage;
- breakdown and mental health problems;
- accidents;
- illness;
- domestic violence;
- risk to children;
- disintegration of family;
- divorce;
- legal battles;
- financial loss and disadvantage;
- self-harm and suicide.

Barriers to adult with Asperger's Syndrome receiving help

- Adults with the characteristics of Asperger's Syndrome can be highly intelligent, even genius. It is not uncommon for adults with Asperger's Syndrome to have highly recognised professional qualifications in fields such as Engineering, Medicine, IT, Science, Accounting, Law, Art, Film, Acting, Photography, Music, Languages, Academia, etc.
- Society assumes consistency of intelligence in all areas of life and therefore has corresponding expectations.
- Adults with Asperger's Syndrome may be eloquent and have strong skills in language and verbal expression but this can be misleading and prevent the detection of underlying difficulties with interpretation and processing, leading to acts of discrimination or injustice against them and their families.
- Adults with Asperger's Syndrome may respond to a situation by withdrawing or by escalating verbally or emotionally. These reactions are typically interpreted as avoidance, obstruction or aggression, when in fact they may be signs of stress, fear, panic, feeling overwhelmed, not knowing what is expected of them or not knowing what to say or do. These reactions could also be an attempt to create distance or regain a sense of control in the midst of confusion and unpredictability. Physical restraint, raising voice or use of force will traumatise a person with Asperger's Syndrome and will further increase barriers to appropriate help being provided.
- May have limited capacity for effective self-advocacy or securing access to other forms of advocacy or legal representation.
- Some behaviours may be incorrectly interpreted as criminal, harmful or obstructive;

Barriers to partner or family members receiving help

- neither they nor the care systems know about Asperger's Syndrome;
- can't adequately describe what is taking place in relationship or family situation and claims may be perceived as implausible;
- adult with Asperger's Syndrome may be able to mask difficulties in public;
- care systems brush off, play down or interpret problems incorrectly;
- appropriate supports and services are simply not available.

Barriers to adult with Asperger's Syndrome seeking help

- limited self-insight so may not recognise the extent of their difficulties;
- limited ability to recognise the impact their difficulties may be having on family members and others;
- fear of failure or being seen as defective;
- an historical experience of not being understood;
- communication and social difficulties may limit access to or compliance with services;
- fear of being bullied, rejected, exploited or discriminated against;
- may not realise that help is available;
- may have developed the belief that others have the problem, not them.

Barriers to partner or family members seeking help

- frustration and anxiety over inability to adequately articulate experiences and needs;
- belief, based on past experiences, that other people including care systems won't believe them and can't help them;
- instinct that family member with Asperger's Syndrome is innocent of intentionally causing harm;
- fear of being judged or punished for failures or mistakes;
- fear of having children removed by child welfare agencies;
- fear of reprisal from adult with Asperger's Syndrome or other family members for revealing family secrets.

Improved awareness within our care systems in relation to Asperger's Syndrome in adult relationships and parenting, and the provision of appropriate supports or referrals, will ensure that families are assisted to re-build the resilience and capacity they began with and enable them to cope better with the circumstances they have been dealt.

How?

Assisting families to re-build the resilience and capacity they began with may be as simple as:

- belief in and support for family members seeking help;
- care systems trained in how to respond and support adults and families appropriately;
- referral to psychological services as needed;
- increasing societal awareness and understanding.

(Extended version of ASPIA Advocacy Leaflet titled "Improved Awareness within Care Systems may help prevent Family Breakdown". Based on Poster prepared for Asia Pacific Autism Conference 2009 (APAC 09). The information contained in this leaflet has been gathered over a period of nine years and is drawn from the testimonials of more than 1000 Australian families. Written by Carol Grigg, Co-Founder and President of ASPIA INC, Asperger Syndrome Partner Information Australia Incorporated. ASPIA has been conducting support group meetings and educational workshops in Sydney since 2003, as well as providing a helpline and website for information. Visit www.aspia.org.au or email info@aspia.org.au .)

Section 6 ASPIA's Story

ASPIA: A Place for Validation, Information, Inspiration

ASPIA INC

A place for . . .

. . . Validation

    . . . Information

        . . . Inspiration

Mutual acknowledgement and understanding of the Asperger marriage experience for partners of adults with (or suspected of having) Asperger's Syndrome.

A sense of belonging ...

"All of us who attend meetings are feeling the benefit of having our own connecting point where we can talk frankly about our struggles and breakthroughs.

It's like finding our own "tribe", like we belong." Carol, Dec 2008/Jan 2009

Our beginnings

The vision to start a support group began in the year 2000 when my own journey into awareness of Asperger's Syndrome began.

I first heard the words "Asperger's Syndrome" in July of that year, and the description seemed to explain the behaviours my own husband was manifesting. I had no idea it was related to Autism, I didn't know what Autism really was anyway, and I had no idea to contact the local Autism Association for information or a referral.

The urgency to find information and advice quickly consumed me and I learned to use the internet. I launched several distressed emails to several websites, one of these being in the UK and the response came back to contact my local Autism Association.

Another website I contacted was the Asperger Syndrome Australian Information Centre run by a wonderful guy named Mitch in South Australia. Mitch conversed with me by email and provided some life-saving answers and a priceless human connection for me. Mitch continues to be a source of encouragement, support and inspiration for me, and he is very supportive of our support group, listing it on his website to help partners find us. I believe it was also during this time that I was made aware of the FAAAS website where much helpful information is provided.

The NSW Autism Association, now known as Autism Spectrum Australia (ASPECT) was able to provide me with the names of several psychologists in Sydney.

In October 2000 we consulted with one of these psychologists, and a very wonderful and supportive connection began and has continued. It was through this psychologist that I was given the opportunity early in 2001 to meet Lyn, whose husband also had Asperger's Syndrome. Lyn and I became firm friends instantly and experienced together those first amazing feelings of validation and relief that come when you finally find someone who knows what you're talking about, who lives through the same experiences and you don't have to try and describe the context or behaviours or suffer the knock-back or minimisation or skepticism or rejection.

Gradually, through an online mailing list and by leaving contact details with the Autism Association, we began to build up a small group which, by early 2003 had grown to around 6. We would meet from time to time and have coffee or picnics and found these times to be like a life-line for us. In May 2003 The Autism Association held a Partner Forum at Macquarie University during Autism Awareness Week. There were about 24 partners in attendance at this forum and we all came away excited and inspired by having been together and shared our experiences. It was at this forum that Anthony Warren of the Autism Association allowed me to announce and launch GRASP, a support group for spouses and partners (and ex-partners). We commenced meetings on 7 June 2003 at Parramatta RSL Club, who allowed us to use the Lachlan Room free of charge. In January 2006, needing a new venue due to larger numbers, we moved our meetings to the College of Nursing at Burwood (NSW).

The idea of a support group was born from those first feelings of desperation at not being able to find someone nearby who understood and could help. A passion began to grow within me to do something to help others, to somehow be or provide a connecting point for others at the beginning of their journeys.

Since our commencement in 2003 the attendance at our meetings has grown from 5 or 6 to an average of 25. Our contact list has grown to around 500. We have regular contributions from a number of excellent Sydney-based psychologists.

Incorporating as an Association had been a dream for a long time, but as a group, and also as individuals, I don't believe we were ready for that step until 2005. There are many things that are possible to achieve from the springboard of being a legal entity.

Our priority, as always, is to continue to provide information and support to those who enquire or attend our meetings, but other priorities involve the need to increase awareness within our general community and urgently among those in the help professions, particularly counsellors, psychologists, doctors and psychiatrists who are often the portal through which many couples and partners seek help and Asperger's Syndrome is not being recognised or identified.

Carol Grigg (October 2005)

Our purpose

General

Our purpose is not to catastrophise the difficulties in an Asperger marriage and bring about its downfall, BUT RATHER to acknowledge the difficulties and differences and provide objective information on how Asperger's Syndrome impacts on a relationship and what steps can be taken to reduce the confusion, conflict and crushing emotional experiences that characterise the private lives of those affected.

We are aware now that over the last few years many partners have been helped by gaining an understanding of Asperger's Syndrome which has enabled them to change their expectations of their partners, themselves and their relationships.

It is also strongly recommended that partners seek help from a professional experienced with Asperger's Syndrome in adults and relationships. There is guidance that can be given in this context that a support group or written information cannot give, and specific characteristics and situations can be addressed.

Meeting and speaking with other partners face-to-face brings an enormous sense of validation for our experiences which can become an invaluable source of strength and inspiration for the task ahead.

Those who've been unable to stay with their relationships testify to finding a place of closure for all their confusion, pain and sense of failure.

The Website

Establishing a website is seen as a way of providing a port of call for partners in Australia and access to helpful information, professionals and supportive contacts.

If you have information, contacts, services, groups or events that you would like us to know about, please contact us.

Listings and advertisements on our website do not automatically indicate our endorsement or promotion of the entire content or views held by those individuals or organisations.

Listings are provided in good faith for the benefit of readers seeking constructive information and support for their personal or professional need.

Dated: 29 October 2005 (Website established)

ASPIA's Aims and Objectives, as provided on our Application for Incorporation as an Association

Our objective:

- To provide supportive information and contacts for partners of adults with Asperger's Syndrome

Our principal activities:

- Answering enquiries
- Providing information and newsletters
- Organising and holding support group meetings and seminars
- Promoting awareness within community about Asperger's Syndrome in adults and marriage.

Dated: 29 July 2005

ASPIA's Constitution and Disclaimer

Asperger Syndrome Partner Information Australia Incorporated (ASPIA INC)

CONSTITUTION

29 July 2005

ASPIA is an organisation run by Partners of Adults with Asperger's Syndrome, for Partners of Adults with Asperger's Syndrome. ("Partners" also includes "Ex-Partners")

Whilst we respect individuals with Asperger's Syndrome, and would welcome and encourage support groups designed for their needs, we declare that ASPIA support group meetings are exclusively for partners & ex-partners of adults with Asperger's Syndrome, and interested or supportive guests from time to time.

The purpose of our organisation as a whole is to provide information on Asperger's Syndrome within marriage/relationships and families and to provide support for partners & ex-partners of individuals with or suspected of having Asperger's Syndrome.

The purpose of our support group meetings is to provide a safe and supportive environment in which partners can debrief, share their concerns openly and honestly with other partners/ex-partners and feel assured of being heard, believed, included, acknowledged, validated, affirmed, encouraged and respected.

Our desire is that partners be encouraged and strengthened to the point where they begin to heal, regain confidence and a sense of self, learn personal boundaries and find a renewed sense of dignity. We believe this can be achieved by meeting with other partners and having the opportunity to receive appropriate information and education in relation to Asperger's Syndrome and marriage/families and also topics relating to coping, boundaries, health issues, personal healing and growth for partners.

We believe that educating and validating partners enables and empowers them to consider options and make informed choices in relation to their future.

Whilst it is our desire to provide all partners with the information, support and assistance they need in order to remain in their marriage or relationship and to cope better, our primary concern is the psychological and physical well-being of the non-Asperger partner.

We encourage all members of ASPIA to take appropriate opportunities outside of our meetings to help spread awareness of Asperger's Syndrome and marriage/families and advocate for our Cause, in as dignified a manner as possible.

We acknowledge that Asperger's Syndrome is a complex disorder involving many characteristics and behaviours in varying degrees. Each partner's experience within marriage will therefore be different, yet similar, with some characteristics manifesting more or less severely from one case to the next. Every partner's experience is valid, and equally difficult to understand and live with.

We commit ourselves and promise each other that we will always remain patient and respectful towards one another, willing to listen and validate in the same way that others listen and validate us.

We will protect the privacy of other members by not sharing anything that would identify other members outside of our meetings.

We commit ourselves to endeavour at all times to be loyal to the aims and objectives of ASPIA as set out above.

Disclaimer

ASPIA is a support group for the sharing of information and experiences. ASPIA does not claim to be providing professional advice to its members and contacts. Whilst all care is taken to share information from reliable sources, ASPIA does not take responsibility for the way this information is implemented in personal situations.

At all times ASPIA encourages partners to seek professional advice relevant to their individual situation from a qualified Practitioner such as a Psychologist, Psychiatrist or Counsellor.

ASPIA INC, Asperger Syndrome Partner Information Australia Incorporated

ABN 30 583 771 917

PO Box 57 Macarthur Square LPO, MACARTHUR NSW 2560

Web: www.aspia.org.au Email: info@aspia.org.au

ASPIA meetings . . . an inside view

ASPIA is a support group and website providing validation and support for partners of adults with Asperger's Syndrome. Even though our support is aimed at non-Asperger partners, we are still part of the general community of support for families affected by Asperger's Syndrome.

We realise that partners with Asperger's Syndrome could fear we are "Aspie bashers" and that we are trying to break up Asperger marriages. By explaining a little about what goes on in our meetings and describing some of the outcomes in the lives of those attending, we hope we can provide some reassurance to those who are concerned.

Those who attend our meetings would be aware that most of the partners attending are looking for ways to stay with their marriages and in the majority of cases they do.

We have sought to bring frequent professional input into our meetings so that partners can learn more about AS, understand their AS partners and find ways to ease the mis-communication and conflict that is a dominant characteristic in their relationship.

We are also building up an excellent library of books that all focus on understanding AS & practical suggestions for a more successful relationship.

For many partners just understanding makes all the difference because they can then make adjustments to their expectations of themselves, their partners and their relationships and live more at peace within that. We see the difference on their faces from one month to the next as they begin to come to terms with their own reality, find ways to respect themselves better and find more effective ways to cope at home.

For some the help has come too late. The long-term confusion, lack of awareness of AS, absence of support and intervention and layers of unresolved issues have all taken too great a toll. The partner has to face the reality that to hold the relationship together any longer could mean the loss of their own emotional and physical health and well-being permanently. In many cases it is the needs of the children that must become the priority, and be balanced against the ongoing effort required to save the struggling marriage.

Some who previously separated have chosen to return to the relationship on new or refreshingly unconventional terms, including partial separation. This may enable them to enjoy "togetherness" in activities that they enjoy, but also to enjoy activities as individuals as well.

Some continue on in the difficult circumstances and are just glad to have our newsletters or a place like our ASPIA meetings to receive validation and be reminded of their own value.

The best situations are where the partner with characteristics of Asperger's Syndrome is willing to accept they have these traits and to co-operate with professional advice and the guidance of their partner. Every non-AS partner would wish for this, and it is the key that would make a beautiful difference in every situation.

Yes, ASPIA meetings are a place for sharing our difficulties but this enables partners to de-brief and receive validation – all in the context of confidentiality and relative anonymity.

Once we have had an opportunity to "get things off our chest" we are then ready and able to take on board the positives of new learning that will help us approach our relationships with renewed energy and hope. Carol Grigg (July 2008)

ASPIA's Unsung Hero ...

In this newsletter (December 2010) I would like to take the opportunity to acknowledge and thank Lyn, ASPIA's Co-Founder, for her tireless commitment to our group, and for her role as my personal "right-hand man" and backstop since we began. Personally she has been a reference point for me all along, an advisor and often an anchor as well.

Lyn is ASPIA Inc's Vice-President, she keeps our Annual General Meetings on track, attends to many details behind the scenes, and on the day of our workshops like the one in October (2010) where we had 220 people in attendance, Lyn oversees the registration table, organises speaker gifts head of time, takes care of all the "on-the-spot" admin and crises on the day, and then the post-event follow up while I collapse. ☺

In February 2011 it will be 10 years since Lyn and I were introduced to each other by our mutual psychologist at the time, Lydia Fegan, who has since retired.

Neither Lyn nor I had previously spoken to any other person who had lived with a partner with Asperger's Syndrome, so our bond is unique and very significant to us. The validation we experienced as we first talked together was truly life-changing.

ASPIA was born from this friendship, and I would like to acknowledge this in this Newsletter. I would also, on behalf of ASPIA, like to congratulate Lyn on her retirement from school teaching at the end of this year, and wish her joy and fulfilment in the exciting new ventures she has planned (as well as staying on with ASPIA!).

Congratulations and thank you Lyn. Carol (December 2010)

Section 7 Establishing a Support Group - Samples and Guides

EIGHT CURATIVE FACTORS OF GROUP

(Benefits of Attending a Support Group)

1. To give FEEDBACK
2. To receive FEEDBACK
3. To offer SUPPORT
4. To receive SUPPORT
5. To recognise that others experience similar difficulties
6. To hear how others resolve problems
7. To offer own ways to solve similar problems
8. To feel ACCEPTED as a group member

Caution is Wise …

Establishing a partner support group is a responsibility that should never be taken lightly.

Particular consideration needs to be made as to the gravity of what we are doing. Marriages, long-term relationships and family units are extremely valuable, even sacred, and may hold more meaning for these partners and family members than anything else they hold dear in their lives. Not only do non-Asperger partners value their marriages, Asperger partners do too, so it is vitally important that the support group undertaking be approached in as positive and constructive a manner as is possible, with strong connections and regular involvement from experienced and mature professionals, particularly psychologists where possible.

Potential support group leaders must have a thorough knowledge of Asperger's Syndrome and a deep understanding of the ways it affects individuals, couples and family situations. Education is vitally important, and potential leaders would be advised to have attended workshops, be widely read, be firmly connected to a network of support already, ideally be a partner or ex-partner themselves and have experienced counselling and psychological guidance for their own situation.

Confidentiality must be stressed at the commencement of every meeting. What is shared in the group stays in the group. No support group can retain its integrity unless this is observed as a matter of utmost importance. See ASPIA's Group Guidelines, this Section.

When partners attend the support group for the first time, they are typically in a state of shell-shock, feeling overwhelmed with new information, the legacy of having lived for years with no validation and a sense of confusion and grief resembling a tidal wave.

Group leaders must establish a warm and accepting environment, and ensure new attendees are quickly connected in with others in attendance.

Sensitivity and caution must be exercised in relation to expecting new attendees to share personal information in the group context before they are ready. Remember they may already be experiencing some trauma, and the last thing we want is for the group experience to be traumatic for them too. Tears or emotional break-down may also cause embarrassment and a reluctance to return to the group. Be sure to reassure group members that tears are ok, and that they are welcome to take a break during the meeting if they need to.

From time to time it has been necessary to remind group members that some attitudes expressed in the meetings are unacceptable. They may be remarks stemming from much grief and bitterness, but negative attitudes can be disturbing to others and it is important to stress consideration and restraint. This is covered in the Group Guidelines.

At all times we remind group members that professional help is recommended additionally to attendance at the support group. An experienced professional can guide a partner carefully and personally in ways that a group context cannot.

We also mention in our group guidelines that attendance at one meeting is not enough to adequately benefit from the group experience. A partner really needs to attend consistently for at least six months and even a year to fully benefit from the educational and support opportunities provided by the group programme and to achieve a more balanced perspective and understanding.

It is not recommended for partners to make any life-changing decisions (unless they are physically or emotionally unsafe at home) until they have gained a thorough understanding of Asperger's Syndrome and how it can be managed in the home. Partners should be encouraged to separate if there is a risk of physical or emotional harm should they remain in the home, or if there is no apparent risk, they should be supported to learn alternative communication techniques that may help to reduce the emotional atmosphere in the home and relationship.

It is recommended to have 4 – 6 educational presentations to the group throughout the year by experienced Psychologists or Educators. This ensures that group members are constantly growing in their understanding of Asperger's Syndrome and keeping up with the latest theories and ideas. Having constructive educational content like this also helps ensure that the group atmosphere remains positive and healthy.

It is also healthy to have a number of informal discussion times throughout the year to enable group members to consolidate their learning and the group experience.

Offering books through a library has also greatly contributed to strengthening the knowledge base of group members.

Carol Grigg, March 2012

Clarifying who ASPIA is for …

ASPIA has always stated clearly that we are a support group for partners of adults with Asperger's Syndrome.

ASPIA cannot meet the support needs of both partners.

In our last ASPIA meeting, ASPIA was described as being like what Al-Anon is to the partners and family members of those who attend AA meetings.

In ASPIA meetings partners have permission to acknowledge the realities and difficulties of being in a relationship with someone with Asperger's Syndrome.

ASPIA meetings are to be a safe place for partners to be validated, informed and inspired.

In ASPIA meetings partners receive information that helps them understand their Asperger partners and the difficulties they are experiencing.

Many partners who have attended ASPIA meetings have been able to become more objective about their expectations of themselves and their partners.

Most partners who attend our meetings experience an improvement in their self-esteem and general well-being.

The Asperger partners of people who attend our meetings will benefit by their partners having a place to be heard and supported and educated.

From time to time ASPIA will hold educational events that are suitable for Asperger people to attend and this will be specifically advertised.

There are other groups and contacts available for people with Asperger's Syndrome.

If you are an adult with Asperger's Syndrome, please refer to our website or contact Autism Spectrum Australia (Sydney) to find support that's appropriate and suitable for your specific needs.

Anyone attending ASPIA meetings is to be prepared to abide by some group rules that stipulate that our agenda is the mutual support of non-Asperger partners.

It is also assumed that those seeking membership of ASPIA support the aims, goals and objectives of ASPIA.

Carol Grigg (June 2007)

A few additional words . . .

When contacting ASPIA please bear in mind that we do not advertise to be providing professional services.

ASPIA is a self-funded incorporated association, run by volunteers, set up to provide information and a support group for partners and family members of adults with Asperger's Syndrome.

ASPIA does not receive any government or non-government funding or sponsorships.

Carol (April 2010)

Typical Meeting Format

ASPIA's Support Group for Partners of Adults with Asperger's Syndrome

- ASPIA's meetings are held monthly on the first Saturday of every month (except January) from 2.00pm – 5.00pm.

A typical meeting would proceed as follows:

- 1.30pm - Set up room, including tables for sign-in and library/literature display
- Set out library books and borrowing sheets
- Place hand-outs on chairs. These state what ASPIA is and what the group guidelines/rules are.
- Welcome Attendees as they arrive.
- Ask Attendees to add their name and email address to the attendance sheet, place contribution in box and write name on an adhesive name tag.
- Newcomers are provided with a hand-out containing information for New Attendees.
- 2.00pm - Mingle & chat with others, have a cuppa and a snack (till approx. 2.30pm)
- 2.30pm - Attendees arc asked to move into the meeting room and take a seat. Chatting continues until the leader commences the meeting.
- A general welcome is given, ad lib comments made, relevant news items are mentioned, then each attendee is asked to briefly introduce themselves and give a little info about what brought them to ASPIA.
- New attendees are welcomed and supported through this, and if any become emotional, an opportunity is made to go into another room and have a chat before they continue with the group session.
- Following this introduction, the group guidelines (as per the hand-out provided on the chairs) are read out by the leader. The group guidelines were brainstormed by the group some years ago and it has been noted that the tone and stability of the meetings have become more positive as a result of this ritual. Reading the guidelines seems to focus and calm everyone ready for mutual and respectful sharing and support.
- If a speaker has been arranged for this meeting, they are introduced next and invited to commence their presentation or topic discussion.
- If there is no speaker arranged, then group discussion follows. Sometimes this will be focused on a chosen topic, sometimes the discussion will be informal and just based on the particular difficulties being faced in the relationship at the time. Shared experiences and ideas can be an extremely valuable resource for group members.
- In recent times, due to attendance numbers and a desire to create a more intimate sharing time, we have been breaking up into small groups of approximately 6 attendees in each group. We may discuss a topic or just chat informally, but the small group idea is proving to be very effective in allowing more people a chance to contribute, especially those who are less confident in a larger group.
- 4.30pm - At this time (approximately) we re-gather the whole group together again to summarise and make any closing comments.
- We then return to the dining area for further refreshments.

During the time before and after the meeting, attendees are given an opportunity to:

- Sign up as financial members of ASPIA
- Borrow books from the library (members only)
- Browse brochures and business cards of recommended professionals
- Pick up a leaflet or newsletter.
- Get to know other group members.

Attendees greatly enjoy the warm and accepting atmosphere of the group and are usually very reluctant to leave. Many good friendships have been made over the years, and many continue to attend over long periods of time. On average we have between 15 – 25 attendees at each meeting, four or five of these being new attendees.

Carol Grigg, 26 March 2012

What is ASPIA?

ASPIA is a support group for:

- Partners of adults with Asperger's Syndrome
- Ex-partners
- Other adults who identify as needing support, information and understanding from the non-Asperger perspective

Our focus is on the needs and issues within an adult relationship, not issues relating to parenting a child with Asperger's Syndrome.

Our meetings were established to bring together individuals with a shared experience who need further insights in order to move forward towards clarity and recovery in his or her personal life.

Our desire is to provide a safe place for these individuals to unburden, find acceptance and an opportunity to discuss issues of concern.

Our goal is that every individual who attends an ASPIA meeting will experience validation and receive information and support that will assist that individual on their journey to:

- recover his or her own sense of self;
- understand Asperger's Syndrome;
- understand the impact Asperger's Syndrome may have had on his or her relationship;
- discover ways to cope better;
- find ideas that may lead to implementing positive change within his or her relationship;
- find closure if the relationship has already ended.

ASPIA INC

www.aspia.org.au

ASPIA Meeting Guide for New Attendees

Asperger Syndrome Partner Information Australia Incorporated

Meeting Guide for New Attendees

Welcome to ASPIA, a support group for partners of adults with Asperger's Syndrome.

Please add your name and email address to the attendance sheet as you enter, place $. . . . in the contribution box and write your name on a name tag.

Help yourself to a cup of tea or coffee in the adjoining kitchen and introduce yourself to others as comfortable. Toilets are just along the corridor near the lifts.

ASPIA is an incorporated association which you are welcome to join for an annual fee of $. . . . if you wish. Application forms are on the side table. Membership entitles you to borrow books from our library, come to meetings for $. . . . , enjoy discounts for workshop events, and be part of our private facebook group and contact list (when available).

Please note that becoming a member of ASPIA is not a requirement for attending meetings or being on the general newsletter email list.

ASPIA has a library which you are welcome to browse but borrowing is for members only.

It is likely that you found us through our website at www.aspia.org.au . If not, please visit our website and become familiar with it. This is a valuable resource for a range of information, and group leaders and speakers tend to assume that attendees are familiar with its content.

ASPIA has some group guidelines, most of which are common to all support groups. These, as well as some more specific information about ASPIA, are set out in a hand-out placed on the chairs in the meeting room.

We hope you will find today's meeting informative and validating. Additional help and support is available from one of the psychologists recommended on our website.

Sincerely,

ASPIA INC

ASPIA Meeting Guidelines / Rules

- Maintain Confidentiality.
- What is heard and said in the group stays within the group.
- If you see a group member in another context outside of this meeting, please do not identify where you know them from.
- Stay with the main group conversation and avoid having side or background conversations at the same time.
- Put phone on silent.
- Be respectful and sensitive towards others in the meeting, even if you don't agree with them.
- Please encourage quiet people to contribute, and avoid monopolising discussions.
- Be aware of your own thoughts and feelings. Shed some tears or take a break if you need to.
- Be careful not to direct any anger at another group member. This creates an unsafe place, and may re-traumatise group members who have come to this meeting to escape an angry or unsafe environment.
- Please refrain from using blatantly derogatory terms or comments in relation to any other person or group of people.
- Be aware that you may leave this meeting with unresolved feelings. Benefits increase as you attend more meetings, and professional help is recommended in addition to attendance at support group meetings.

ASPIA INC

www.aspia.org.au

Section 8 Concluding Thoughts

Essay: Asperger's Syndrome in Relationships - Is there Hope?

It is difficult to write about the realities of relationships affected by Asperger's Syndrome without risking offence to people with Asperger's Syndrome.

It is important however to pause a moment and focus on the reasons for writing about relationships affected by Asperger's Syndrome and why there is such a need for information and validation for all parties concerned.

The reasons for writing about relationships affected by Asperger's Syndrome are because these relationships are confusing and difficult and can involve great stress, grief and trauma for both partners, and any children of the relationship.

Different cultures

The reality is that the person with Asperger's Syndrome and the person without Asperger's Syndrome are as different from each other as people from completely different cultures. We may look the same from the outside, but underneath we are driven by completely different priorities, needs and perceptions. It's deeper than just the differences that normal relationships struggle with.

Whilst it is evident that many people with Asperger's Syndrome do desire to be in relationship and enjoy social situations, it would seem that this is not a priority for them in the same way that it is for people who do not have Asperger's Syndrome.

People with Asperger's Syndrome generally seem to approach things with a system or formula and be more focused on a particular interest, project or task than on relationship with the people around them. For people who do not have Asperger's Syndrome, their relationships are their life-blood and all interests are undertaken in the context of social connectedness in some way.

Immediately this displays the chasm between the two worlds or cultures and goes a long way to explaining the difficulties, strain and unhappiness that characterise most relationships formed between someone who does have Asperger's Syndrome and someone who does not have Asperger's Syndrome.

Who's to blame?

Rather than assigning blame either way, perhaps it is helpful to just begin to adopt the attitude that it's completely understandable that the two worlds are scarcely compatible. It's not about defect. The majority of people with Asperger's Syndrome are enormously gifted in specific fields so they're not inferior. The problem begins because people from the two cultures, namely Asperger and non-Asperger, form a relationship and expect to forge a solid, mutually satisfying conventional marriage relationship. Asperger's Syndrome creates problems in relationship particularly because the person with Asperger's Syndrome does not have the same relational needs as the non-Asperger partner and he or she is mostly unable to instinctively recognise or meet the emotional needs of his or her partner.

Do we give up?

Does this mean that people who have Asperger's Syndrome should not form marriage relationships with people who don't have Asperger's Syndrome? Should those who are already married face the reality and give up?

My experience in support work with partners indicates that there are countless marriages in serious trouble because they haven't had knowledge of Asperger's Syndrome in time to avoid forming seriously dysfunctional relationship patterns. These dysfunctional patterns daily threaten to destroy the relationship and both partners, particularly the non-Asperger partner. How many more marriages are still "in the dark" about the presence of Asperger's Syndrome in their situation? How many marriages have already been lost, and to this day the partners have no idea that the difficulties were caused by the characteristics of Asperger's Syndrome?

Perhaps Asperger's Syndrome in its most honest and purest form is quite amenable. Perhaps it is the denial, the complex and multi-layered coping mechanisms and defensive strategies that make Asperger's Syndrome so difficult to live successfully in relationship with.

Normal expectations of marriage

People who do not have Asperger's Syndrome enter a marriage with the normal expectation that the marriage relationship will be the priority and will be about togetherness, mutual terms and meeting of needs. From the stories I have heard it seems that people with Asperger's Syndrome also have this expectation, at least in theory, but countless testimonies indicate that in reality by some process of attrition the relationship ends up being more one of practicality and convenience for the person with Asperger's Syndrome than for the loving and meeting of emotional needs of the marital partner.

A sentiment expressed by some non-Asperger partners is that they feel their Asperger partner must have analysed them prior to marriage and assessed them as being capable of filling a compensatory role for his or her own social, relational and functional deficits. The non-Asperger partner unwittingly becomes the social bridge and interpreter and often fills the role of personal assistant. In the privacy of their relationship, the person who does not have Asperger's Syndrome will more than likely be physically and emotionally drained, working overtime to mediate relationships for his or her partner and keep life on track for both of them. Perhaps the relationship has taken on more of the characteristics of a business partnership or arrangement.

For those who had normal expectations of the mutuality of marriage, there will be bitter disappointment, a sense of betrayal and a feeling of being used and trapped. Instinctively they know that their partner needs them to carry out these vital roles for them, but feelings develop that the relationship is about the needs and interests of the person with Asperger's Syndrome and that there is not even room for their own needs.

It is these sentiments that set up the hostility expressed by non-Asperger people towards those who have Asperger's Syndrome. Many partners feel that they are daily sacrificing their own values and losing their own souls and sense of self to help fulfill the priorities of the partner who has Asperger's Syndrome. They begin to feel that they have lost their individuality and identity and are entirely defined by the role they fill for their Asperger partner. There's a sense that there is no mutuality, no equality, no justice, no hope.

What is the answer? Is there hope?

I see the only hope for relationship as being contained within the willingness of the person with Asperger's Syndrome to gain as much insight as possible into the realities of his or her differences, recognise the impact this has on his or her relationship, seek professional guidance and co-operate with his or her partner to develop a more healthy mutuality in the relationship. Surely this has to be a condition of entering marriage or continuing in an already established marriage. "How can two walk together except they be agreed?" (Biblical quote)

Ignorance of Asperger's Syndrome

So how do we move on from the impasse that still exists between the two communities? I believe most of this is caused by the ignorance of Asperger's Syndrome that still exists within our communities and professional services. No-one knows enough about it to be able to identify it when they are confronted by it and very few have an adequate understanding of it. Those with Asperger's Syndrome are afraid of being labelled or seen as defective. Those who realise they are living with someone who has it are either disbelieved or crushed by the lack of support and professional help.

People with Asperger's Syndrome can tend to be militant and hold rigidly to what defines them as individuals. They can be very interesting and often likably eccentric. They may have a tendency to claim victimisation from those who do not have Asperger's Syndrome, while they determinedly continue to navigate life and relationships on terms of their own rather than mutuality and compromise. People who do not have Asperger's Syndrome continue to long for the mutual meeting of emotional needs within the marriage and resent the reality of living on terms dictated by the needs and priorities of the partner with Asperger's Syndrome. In effect, their flexibility is exploited by the inflexibility of the person with Asperger's Syndrome.

Of course marriage should not be exclusive to those who do not have Asperger's Syndrome.

However, in the same way that any individual on this earth is responsible to gain self-insight and work on character defects that impact on their relationships (if they wish to stay in a relationship!), so also is the person with Asperger's Syndrome responsible to gain self-insight and work on defects that impact on their relationships. The differences and deficits may be part and parcel of Asperger's Syndrome, but marriage is about both partners taking responsibility for the well-being of the relationship and each other's emotional needs.

If a person with Asperger's Syndrome can't promise the mutuality, relationship and personal sacrifice that is a reasonable expectation within a marriage, then marriage may not be for them. If they are already married, then the least they can offer their partner is honesty and co-operation to find more mutual terms.

Most of the non-Asperger partners I've met are genuinely looking for reasons to stay with their Asperger partners, not leave them. They are looking for strategies and pathways that will ease the conflict and stress points and enable the relationship to improve. From the stories shared in our support group we have learned that some relationships can be improved by the partners negotiating terms and trade-offs and even partial separation (maybe still under the same roof).

I often wish I could personally meet with all the Asperger partners represented by our group and somehow convey to them how loyal their partners are, how hopeful they continue to be that the relationship can be improved and what positive contribution they can have to this process.

Sadly, so many partners with Asperger's Syndrome remain in denial about their Asperger characteristics and the negative contribution they are having in their relationship. They don't seem to have realised that the truth can actually make us free – free to grow, free to heal, free to live, free to love in whatever way we are capable, even if this involves a slightly unconventional approach. Denial is self-defeating and puts a brick on the entire relationship, threatening its very survival.

Carol Grigg

Essay: That Elusive Potential

I am amazed at the human capacity to endure pain, difficulty and crisis in life, and to keep hanging in there, holding on to every thread of hope and trying to make the best of a situation. There is always so much at stake, and so much to lose for everyone concerned, and it is so hard to give up on something that presents with so much promise and so much potential.

It is my experience and observation that this is particularly so when experiencing a difficult marriage and nothing "normal" seems to work. To the last breath so many can remain hopeful and determined that they'll find the answer, "tomorrow will be better", "I'll work out what it is that's causing the problems", "I'll try another approach", "I'll break the code" and then we can get on with the life we dreamed of, together. Instinctively we seem to sense there must be a key and that if only we can find the key … we'll unlock the mystery of what's going wrong between us.

We know there is amazing potential in the relationship, in both partners. We saw this in the beginning. We believed in it. All the facts pointed to so many possibilities – we thought we could soar. Our partners are intelligent, interesting, so gifted, so refreshing. They have the most amazing knowledge about interesting topics and seem to be able to speak on them with so much confidence. They have passions about issues that really matter, their belief systems are strong and clear-cut, they like to do things "right", their sense of logic gives us confidence in their common sense approach to life.

We're the kind of people who celebrate difference and who like to encourage those who may seem on the fringe or gifted in a way that's different. We believe their "differentness" can make an interesting contribution that will decorate the ordinariness of "normal" and bring colourful dimensions to life. We're intrigued by their strong sense of self and purpose, and applaud this. We overlook their quirkiness or eccentricity as just part of their colourful outlook that makes them so gifted and so interesting. We want to be with them, to enjoy them, to soak in what they are to enhance our own lives and we're delighted to feel we can enhance their lives too with the skills we bring to the relationship, particularly in social situations.

Courtship is so ideal. Almost textbook like. We're showered with attention and adulation. The flowers come at the right time, the cards with awkward but deep-feeling words. We feel adored, we're told they're becoming "fond of us". Quaint, but so genuine. We're romanced and feel like we're the luckiest person on the earth at being noticed and chosen by this amazing, interesting though sometimes mysterious person, and to top it off, even though physical appearance is not a priority for us, they're often quite good looking or have a certain charisma. How lucky are we?

Something we have no idea of at the time is just how much we are taking for granted. Worlds of stuff. We are so unsuspecting because we are so "typical" in our thinking and so naïve and idealistic, as is typical for that stage of our lives. We have this in-built assumption that everyone has the same basic approach to everyday stuff including relationships. We believe that even though every person is different and has had different upbringings and childhood pain, psychologically we all still approach things or respond to things in generally the same way. Our whole society seems to be built on this assumption and on conformity to certain unspoken standards and expectations. Most people we know seem to automatically know how to keep their places and make appropriate contributions to life and society at the right times.

This person we've met just seems so refreshing, so different and therefore so capable of potentially contributing even more than the ordinary person. We dream of a very interesting and exciting future together that could leave a special legacy of purpose and achievement, positively influencing the lives of our children and others we connect with along the way.

Our inbuilt flexibility enables us to allow for difference in those around us, but even in this flexibility we are still holding many assumptions and prescribed expectations about how those who are different should behave in any given situation.

One assumption we all hold is that people who are highly intelligent have corresponding levels of common sense and social skills for their intelligence, and our confusion really kicks in when the incongruence starts to become apparent, often after marriage. We have no place in our finite understanding for how this can be, so we automatically assume that character flaws are to blame and we begin to belittle and criticise them for letting us down, even accusing them of tricking us or pretending before the wedding, little realising how unmerciful this really is.

It's at this point we realise that our commitment to share a future together is beginning to go horribly wrong, in ways we just do not understand and don't seem to be able to arrest or address.

I actually don't think anyone in today's society is adequately prepared for the reality of forging a co-operative and successful long-term committed relationship, whether "typical" or "different", although some do seem to develop the skills to make it through successfully. We are deceived by the romanticism of movies, the euphoria of infatuation and over-inflated estimation of our own competence, expecting to live "happily ever after" if we follow the script, but the statistics of failed marriages prove that very few of us are really equipped with the necessary components of respect, emotional maturity and solid communication and negotiation skills to build and sustain that elusive "marital bliss".

For those of us who marry someone "different" we have no idea that we've entered a world for which we've had no chance of being adequately prepared for, and sadly we flounder in a context of bewilderment and ineffectiveness in every way. It's not really any different for the person who is different. They too flounder in a context of expectations that bring their own bewilderment, having no consistency, order or predictability in this puzzling arrangement called marriage.

Many of us find ourselves caught in a place of disillusionment, with the realisation of our hopes and potential as far away as ever.

They say it takes two to tango, and that there is always fault on both sides when a relationship fails. In principle this is true, but I do believe that a relationship can be crippled when the needs and preferences of one partner are regularly prioritised over the needs and preferences of the other partner.

It doesn't take much to imagine how one partner in the equation could end up flourishing while the other begins to languish as their own needs are all too often minimised or denied. Marriage is only truly successful when both partners are committed to caring about and prioritising their partner's needs and person above their own. It has to be mutual to avoid inequality and injustice.

Then the relationship has all the potential in the world. Carol Grigg

Essay: When Hope Fades

It has been more than eleven years now since the Author first heard the words "Asperger's Syndrome" and the journey of learning and understanding was first embarked upon. First one partner, Lyn, joined me, then another, Alison, then Annette, Kathryn and Ruth, and then one by one over the years that followed, both in our meetings and through our website, a throng began to gather to the point where thousands of partners and families have now taken hold of our gesture of support as an anchor in the midst of their turbulence and as a decipherer of the confusion that reigned in the home.

Some of us have attended countless workshops and support group meetings, read every book on the topic, explored every website and generally discussed every angle of Asperger relationships and every avenue of navigation within Asperger relationships with others who are captivated by the same heart-rending desperation to grasp some comprehension of this "difference" of human experience, perception and expression that so stealthily outwits our "typical" expectations and needs within relationship.

No matter how much information any of us have, we come back every time to the personal place in every relationship where partner meets partner, where the challenge to learn, understand, trust, co-operate and adjust is either attempted or evaded.

Essential to every couple's pathway forward is understanding and the acceptance of reality. Both partners must learn about Asperger's Syndrome and ideally have professional guidance.

The non-Asperger partner must accept that Asperger's Syndrome will set the landscape for the future of the relationship, and they must be able to do this without bitterness of heart, or the compulsion to use denigrating words and gestures directed at their partner's "difference" and vulnerabilities.

The Asperger partner must accept and explore the presence of the Asperger characteristics and be willing to accept and respect their partner's desire and need for relationship. Workable methods of communication must be found, conflict must be addressed constructively and emotional escalation within the relationship and home must be brought under control, perhaps with the help of therapies that psychologists can assist with.

There is clearly evidence these days that many adults with Asperger's Syndrome are openly acknowledging their difficulties and responsibly seeking help and knowledge to manage the characteristics that negatively affect their relationships and family life.

ASPIA's experience provides evidence that countless non-Asperger partners are also seeking knowledge and support to recover and re-build their relationships and family life. In fact, if motivation could move mountains, the partners who've attended ASPIA's meetings over the last eight years would have moved the Great Dividing Range into the Pacific Ocean by now!

Our primary relationships are where we invest our hearts, minds, souls and bodies into what we hold the most precious in life. This is the family context into which we bring our children, and share the most special moments. It is heart-breaking and traumatic to be unable to stop the relationship slipping away, in spite of great effort.

Sadly, the majority of the Asperger adults that are in relationships with the non-Asperger partners we support are only making minimal or occasional gestures and attempts in the relationship, at best. For some, this may actually be all they can achieve. Others can achieve greater relationship quality but lack the motivation to give it the same priority that they give other interests in their lives.

Many still lack the will or the insight to acknowledge their Asperger characteristics, and may either stonewall a partner's efforts to communicate or negotiate, or they may aggressively shut-down the partner's efforts.

In other situations, the difference in perception and meaning, and the unresolved misunderstandings these create between partners has sadly led to the Asperger partner building up false beliefs about their partner and his/her motives. It seems that these beliefs often cannot be dismantled, even with the benefit of knowledge, professional help and an opportunity to re-visit those misunderstandings for clarification. These false beliefs have undermined trust and prevent any bridge of communication being reconstructed.

I believe there comes a time when a partner must stand still and begin to weigh up the wisdom of allowing the relationship to continue. If effort has been made to learn and seek support, and adequate time has been given to allow the processes of change to take place, and yet every day events are still compounding the stress and conflict that the partner is trying to overcome, it may be time to respectfully bring the relationship to an end.

Our Asperger partners may have a "difference" that impairs their ability to reciprocate adequately in the relationship, but we, the non-Asperger partners, are still mere humans, and our strengths and abilities are finite. It is vitally important to retain enough emotional and physical strength to be able to continue with life itself, and the ongoing responsibilities of parenting, family life, employment and community participation, etc.

Every month we welcome partners into our group who are shattered in spirit, disempowered in soul and burdened with a palpable grief for the relationship they treasure but can't nourish or be nourished by. There is no magic wand, just human spirit meeting human spirit in a place where burdens are shared with warmth and understanding. If this is a place where knowledge can be gained, and strength re-gathered for the task at hand then we will have fulfilled our purpose of partner support which is reflected in the following words read at the beginning of every support group meeting:

"Our meetings were established to bring together individuals with a shared experience who need further insights in order to move forward towards clarity and recovery in his or her personal life.

Our desire is to provide a safe place for these individuals to unburden, find acceptance and an opportunity to discuss issues of concern.

Our goal is that every individual who attends an ASPIA meeting will experience validation and receive information and support that will assist that individual on their journey to:

- recover his or her own sense of self;
- understand Asperger's Syndrome;
- understand the impact Asperger's Syndrome may have had on his or her relationship;
- discover ways to cope better;
- find ideas that may lead to implementing positive change within his or her relationship;
- find closure if the relationship has already ended."

Carol Grigg, 2 April 2012

ASPIA INC, www.aspia.org.au

For up-to-date support group and referral information, as well as other useful links in relation to Asperger's Syndrome in adults and relationships, please visit:

- ASPIA's website at www.aspia.org.au

- Tony Attwood's website at http://www.tonyattwood.com.au

- or contact your local Autism/Asperger support organisation.

Printed in Great Britain
by Amazon